HEMORRHOIDS

Foods, Supplements & Herbs

Isabel M. Rivero

COPYRIGHT & CREDITS

HEMORRHOIDS. Foods, Supplements & Herbs
Copyright ©2018, 2024 *by* Isabel M. Rivero
All rights reserved

Cover design: Desirée Mendoza M.
Photographs by Buntysmum and Imagemo via Pixabay

This book provides general information and is not a substitute for professional medical advice. Neither the publisher nor the author shall be held liable for any damages of any kind arising from the use of this content. Readers assume full responsibility for their decisions, actions, and outcomes.

This book is intended as a reference only and should never be used as a medical manual. Its purpose is to help readers make informed decisions about their health. It is not intended to replace any treatment prescribed by a doctor.

Original title: *HEMORROIDES. Alimentos y Plantas Medicinales* © 2018, Isabel M. Rivero. All Rights Reserved
© 2024 translated by Laura Mendoza & Sara I. Afonso

Prologue: A Guide to Wellness

Dear Readers,

Welcome to this journey toward better health! Since I began sharing my knowledge and experience, my primary motivation has been to make a positive contribution to your lives. That's why, through these pages, I aim to offer valuable information and practical resources that can genuinely help you feel better.

In this book, every piece of advice and remedy has been thoughtfully chosen for its proven effectiveness and practicality in everyday life. You will discover not only medicinal plants, supplements, and accessible foods but also detailed medical insights into this health concern, along with additional tips and answers to the most frequently asked questions–providing you with a practical, comprehensive, and trustworthy guide.

My goal is for this work to be your valuable and practical companion–a resource where you can find tangible tools to support you on your journey toward a healthier, more fulfilling life. Knowing that this work has a positive impact brings me great joy and motivates me to keep going. While writing requires effort, time, and perseverance, the knowledge that my books make a meaningful difference in your lives is my greatest reward.

Because your experiences are my greatest source of inspiration, I would love for you to write to me and share your progress. Feel free to share your progress by writing directly to me at **isabelmriveror@gmail.com**. Your stories inspire me and truly make my efforts worthwhile.

I sincerely hope this practical guide becomes your indispensable pillar on your journey to better health and well-being. Thank you for allowing me to be part of your life.

With love,

Isabel

INTRODUCTION

On our journey towards achieving optimal health, it's crucial to recognize one fundamental truth: no single "miracle" solution—be it a medication, herb, supplement, or food—can fully resolve an illness on its own. Solely focusing on managing symptoms, while neglecting the deeper "root cause," not only delays true healing but also increases the likelihood of recurrence. Instead, addressing the underlying cause of the problem can lead to a gradual reduction in symptoms and support genuine, long-lasting recovery.

You may have experienced times when treatments or medications didn't seem to deliver the results you had hoped for. This often occurs because restoring health requires a holistic approach—one that goes beyond surface-level treatment to target the root cause of the issue. Effective healing involves more than just the right therapies; it must also encompass vital changes. A well-rounded plan should include improvements to diet (the cornerstone of cellular health), enhanced sleep quality, better stress management, and the cultivation of healthier daily lifestyle habits. Together, these elements strengthen the body's resilience, boost confidence in recovery, and reinforce its natural ability to heal.

This book takes you on a journey through this integrative approach to health and recovery. In the first chapter, we'll provide you with accessible, straightforward explanations of the main causes behind this particular illness. Additionally, we'll cover its key symptoms, variations, early warning signs, potential complications, practical advice to manage them, and the essential medical tests necessary for an accurate diagnosis. This foundation sets the stage for understanding your condition and equips you with the tools needed to address it effectively.

As the chapters unfold, you'll discover practical, evidence-based strategies designed to support your recovery. These include detailed dietary recommendations, easy-to-follow meal plans tailored to your needs, and natural approaches such as supplements and herbal remedies that support gradual, sustained improvement. The guidance provided is both flexible and adaptable, allowing you to choose what works best for your unique health journey.

For those seeking a clear roadmap, the chapter titled "**Suggested Practical Plan**" serves as a comprehensive guide. This section consolidates the most important elements of recovery into an actionable framework, while also pointing you toward additional chapters for deeper insights and tailored advice. By using this plan as your foundation, you'll gain clarity and confidence in navigating the steps toward healing.

It's worth stressing that the guidance in this book is not based on subjective opinions or anecdotal evidence. Rather, every recommendation is supported by scientific research and validated by credible studies. To further reassure you, we've included a comprehensive list of references and studies at the end of the book. This ensures you can trust the methods and feel secure when implementing these strategies into your life.

Through a blend of understanding, practical tips, and scientifically-backed solutions, this book aims to empower you as you work toward true recovery and lasting wellness.

HEMORRHOIDS

The condition commonly known as hemorrhoids, often referred to as piles, is one of the most widespread health issues, touching the lives of millions across all age groups and cultures. Though they can be uncomfortable and even painful at times, the good news is that these instances are rarely dangerous. Better yet, with the advanced treatments available today combined with simple lifestyle adjustments, managing symptoms and achieving a full recovery is completely within reach.

Gaining a deeper understanding of this condition, along with the factors that contribute to its onset, is an essential first step toward successfully addressing it and enhancing your overall quality of life. Hemorrhoids occur when the veins in the anal and rectal areas become swollen or inflamed. They are generally divided into two categories based on their location: internal hemorrhoids, which are often harder to detect in early stages, and external hemorrhoids, which are more visible and tend to cause greater discomfort.

Internal hemorrhoids are located within the rectum, beyond the visible area, as they sit above an anatomical boundary known as the pectinate line. These are part of the submucosal tissues, which, when inflamed, develop into small vascular pads or cushions. Early symptoms might include mild bleeding during bowel movements, typically without pain, as the area has very few nerve endings. However, as the condition progresses, the swollen tissues may protrude from the anal canal, causing increased irritation and discomfort.

External hemorrhoids, on the other hand, are positioned just beneath the skin around the anus, making them visible and often painful. This type of hemorrhoid can swell significantly, sometimes to the point where everyday activities such as sitting or walking become quite challenging. Habitual issues such as constipation, excessive straining during bowel movements, pregnancy, or a diet low in fiber often contribute to their development. Additionally, extended periods of sitting, sedentary lifestyles, and even stress have been identified as common triggers for this type.

In general, both types of hemorrhoids result from increased

pressure within the veins of the affected area. This heightened pressure can arise from factors like straining on the toilet, prolonged sitting, or impaired blood flow, all of which weaken vein walls and lead to inflammation. Other factors, such as genetic predisposition, obesity, high alcohol consumption, aging, and certain medical conditions, can also increase susceptibility.

External hemorrhoids may occasionally develop complications due to clot formation, known as thrombosis. This can lead to severe pain, pronounced swelling, and the appearance of dense, hardened lumps near the anus, which can understandably cause significant distress for those experiencing this condition. Thankfully, with timely and appropriate medical attention, these cases are often resolved relatively quickly, with relief from both pain and swelling.

The body's response varies depending on the type of hemorrhoids present. For internal hemorrhoids, the veins weaken as they lose the support of the surrounding tissues, allowing them to bulge outward from their normal position. In contrast, external hemorrhoids, situated in a more nerve-rich area, are typically accompanied by heightened sensitivity and soreness.

Symptoms largely depend on the location of the hemorrhoids. Internal hemorrhoids are more likely to cause painless bleeding, while external hemorrhoids tend to result in persistent itching, significant discomfort, and challenges in performing everyday activities. Fortunately, a variety of effective treatments are available, ranging from at-home remedies to minimally invasive medical procedures.

Simple lifestyle changes, such as incorporating more dietary fiber into your meals, staying properly hydrated, avoiding prolonged bathroom sessions, and maintaining a regular physical activity routine, can lead to truly remarkable improvements. In addition to these habits, there are numerous treatment options to explore.

If you're struggling with hemorrhoids, take heart: you are not alone. This condition is incredibly common, and the most encouraging part is that it's highly manageable. With the right knowledge, proactive steps, and proper guidance, you can significantly ease your discomfort and regain control of your well-being. This book is here to support you every step of the way, offering valuable insights into the causes, treatments, and lifestyle adjustments that can make a real difference. Beyond just addressing the symptoms, you'll discover practical advice, complementary remedies, and natural solutions to help you feel confident in your path to recovery. Remember, taking the first step toward understanding and managing your condition is already a sign of progress!

Symptoms

The symptoms associated with hemorrhoids can present themselves in various ways, depending on both the type and severity of the condition. Below is a list of the most common symptoms typically linked to this health issue, designed to help you identify them clearly and promptly:

▸ **Rectal bleeding:**
Rectal bleeding is one of the most common and characteristic symptoms of hemorrhoids. During bowel movements, bright red blood may appear, typically coating the stool, staining toilet paper, or showing as a thin stream that leaves marks in the toilet. It is important to note that, in the case of hemorrhoids, the blood does not mix directly with the stool.

While rectal bleeding is never considered normal, it is not always indicative of the severity of hemorrhoids. Some individuals may bleed due to fragile skin, while others, even with larger or more advanced hemorrhoids, may not experience this symptom. The amount of blood also varies; it may range from a few drops to heavier bleeding. Typically, this bleeding lasts a few days, subsides, and may recur weeks or months later. Generally, it does not occur between bowel movements unless an internal hemorrhoid prolapses or extends outside the anus.

Certain factors, such as wearing tight clothing–especially jeans –can exacerbate external hemorrhoids, potentially causing ulcers due to constant friction in the affected area.

If bleeding occurs almost daily, persists for more than five days, or becomes excessively heavy, consulting a doctor is essential. Prolonged bleeding can lead to anemia and may signal a more serious condition, such as colon or rectal cancer. In these cases, the blood often mixes with the stool and tends to appear darker in color. Seeking medical attention promptly ensures timely diagnosis and treatment, increasing the likelihood of a favorable outcome.

▸ **Pain or discomfort:**
In general, uncomplicated hemorrhoids do not cause pain. At

most, they may create a sensation of heaviness or pressure in the lower rectum. However, pain typically occurs only when complications arise, such as thrombosis, infections, ulcerations, fissures, abscesses, papillitis, or cryptitis, among others.

Pain that begins 15 to 20 minutes after a bowel movement, gradually intensifies, lasts for several hours, subsides, and then recurs with subsequent bowel movements likely indicates the presence of an anal fissure. On the other hand, if the pain appears suddenly, is constant, persists through the night, and subsides after one or two days, accompanied by a lump at the anus, it may suggest hemorrhoidal thrombosis. This condition occurs when a vein becomes blocked due to the formation of a blood clot.

If the pain resembles that of thrombosis but is accompanied by fever and general discomfort, it could indicate a rectal abscess, which involves the accumulation of pus within the affected area. Occasionally, a complication known as a "hemorrhoidal crisis" may also occur, where hemorrhoids become severely inflamed without thrombosis. This results in ongoing rectal discomfort, a persistent sensation of swelling, a feeling as though a foreign object is present, or the sensation of incomplete bowel evacuation. This type of pain worsens during bowel movements and may also cause discomfort while walking.

Although anal pain could, in rare cases, be associated with anal cancer, rectal cancer typically does not cause pain in its early stages. Seeking medical attention in cases of uncertainty is essential.

The pain associated with hemorrhoids can range from mild discomfort or pressure to sharp and intense pain. In most cases, it is linked to external hemorrhoids, as the dilated veins are easily irritated from friction during everyday activities such as walking, sitting, or passing stool. When thrombosed hemorrhoids are present, the pain can be particularly severe due to the pressure caused by the blood clot.

▸ **Itching and irritation:**
The skin around the anus can become irritated and itchy due to contact with hemorrhoids. The intensity of this sensation can vary, ranging from mild to severe, and may create a tingling sensation or an uncontrollable urge to scratch. Itching is often more pronounced when lying down or during the night.

This itching can persist for days, weeks, or even months,

alternating between periods of improvement and worsening. Over time, the episodes of itching may last longer, with shorter intervals of relief.

If left untreated, the irritation and itching can spread beyond the anus, affecting areas such as the vagina and perineum in women, or the groin, the crease between the buttocks, the thighs, and the base of the penis in men.

The primary cause of this itching is moisture caused by anal discharge, which is associated with several factors:

> *Protruding hemorrhoids*: These are often accompanied by rectal mucosa that moistens the surrounding skin.

> *Large hemorrhoids*: Instead of bleeding, they may produce increased amounts of discharge. When combined with gases, this moisture can irritate the skin.

> *Small hemorrhoids with weak anal muscles*: This combination can lead to persistent moisture in the area.

> *Excessive or improper hygiene*: Frequent washing, prolonged sitz baths, or failing to properly dry the area often leaves it damp for long periods, which can aggravate itching.

> **Prolapse:**
In some cases, internal hemorrhoids may prolapse, meaning they slip out of the anal canal during bowel movements or even while at rest. Prolapse typically occurs during defecation, and for individuals without medical training, it can be difficult to distinguish whether the lumps felt during hygiene practices are external clots, inflamed external hemorrhoids, prolapsed internal hemorrhoids, a protruding tumor, or rectal prolapse. For this reason, it is essential to seek medical advice for an accurate diagnosis.

When trying to identify the origin of lumps around the anus, the following characteristics can serve as initial guidance:

> *Prolapsed internal hemorrhoids*: These appear as soft, reddish lumps. Generally, they are not painful, may retract on their own or with manual assistance, and typically appear during defecation. In some cases, however, they may remain outside the anus.

> *Thrombosis*: These lumps are purplish in color, firm in

texture, and usually accompanied by significant pain.

‣ *Fibroma or anal fissure*: Characterized by intense pain that begins 15 to 20 minutes after bowel movements, diminishes after 6 to 9 hours, and recurs under similar circumstances the following day.

‣ *Abscess*: These lumps are poorly defined, associated with constant pain, and are often accompanied by fever.

‣ *Exteriorized polyp or tumor*: These present as very hard, reddish lumps that may bleed but are generally not painful. It is crucial to consult a doctor promptly, as this could be an early sign of cancer.

In addition to occurring during bowel movements, hemorrhoids may also prolapse following intense physical exertion or prolonged standing. In the early stages, prolapsed hemorrhoids often retract spontaneously into the anal canal. However, over time–months or even years–it may become necessary to manually reposition them.

To manually reposition hemorrhoids, it is helpful to lie on your back, relax, bend your knees, and keep your legs slightly apart while gently pushing them back into place. In more advanced cases, applying pressure with the entire hand may be required to stabilize them.

On the other hand, external hemorrhoids can become strangulated due to a spasm of the anal sphincter. This may result in blood within them clotting, causing significant inflammation and severe pain. If left untreated, this condition can develop into a more serious clinical scenario, marked by excruciating pain that may become unbearable and resistant to all forms of medication, requiring surgical intervention.

‣ **Feeling of Fullness or Pressure**:
Many individuals may feel a sensation of fullness, pressure, or heaviness in the anal area as a result of hemorrhoids. This sensation can be uncomfortable and, in some cases, may worsen after extended periods of sitting or after bowel movements.

‣ **Discomfort During Bowel Movements**:
Hemorrhoids can make bowel movements more difficult. This difficulty arises from a sensation of obstruction or blockage caused by inflammation in the area, resulting in discomfort during defecation.

‣ **Sensation of a Lump or Mass in the Anal Area:**
Prolapsed hemorrhoids, especially external ones, often appear as noticeable lumps or masses in the anal area. These lumps may be sensitive to touch, leading to pain or discomfort when sitting or during bowel movements.

‣ **Fecal or Mucus Leakage:**
In some cases, hemorrhoids may cause involuntary leakage of stool or mucus. This occurs as a result of irritation and inflammation in the anal area, which is more common when the hemorrhoids are prolapsed or when additional infections or irritations are present.

‣ **Sensitivity to Touch or Friction:**
Painful and inflamed hemorrhoids can become highly sensitive to contact. Actions such as wiping after using the toilet or sitting may be particularly uncomfortable or painful due to friction affecting the irritated area.

‣ **Tenesmus:**
The term "tenesmus" describes the persistent, uncomfortable sensation of needing to defecate, even when bowel movements feel incomplete or nothing is expelled. This occurs because the rectum lacks nerve endings that detect pain but does have nerves that sense heat and cold. Additionally, pressure-sensitive nerve endings in the rectum are responsible for generating the sensation of fullness, which leads to repeated urges to defecate.

‣ **Soiling:**
In Grade III and IV hemorrhoids, soiling may occur as a result of mucus secretion. This mucus, combined with the presence of protruding anal lumps, can make maintaining proper hygiene in the affected area difficult, often resulting in stains on underwear. This condition can be uncomfortable and serves as a key indicator for the need to treat hemorrhoids effectively to prevent further complications.

It is crucial to note that symptoms associated with hemorrhoids can vary widely among individuals, depending on factors such as the severity of the condition, lifestyle, diet, and the presence of other underlying health issues. Moreover, some individuals may experience only mild symptoms or may even remain asymptomatic, which can complicate the diagnosis and delay proper identification.

Types of Hemorrhoids

Hemorrhoids are classified into two main types: internal and external. This classification is based on their anatomical location, with each type exhibiting distinct characteristics and symptoms. Below, we'll take a closer look at the unique features of each type to help you gain a better understanding of this condition.

MAIN TYPES OF HEMORRHOIDS

▸ **Internal Hemorrhoids**: These form inside the rectum, above the dentate line–an area where the lining of the large intestine transitions to the skin of the anal region. Internal hemorrhoids are typically less painful than external ones because they are not exposed to direct friction. Although usually not visible, they can produce symptoms such as:

▸ *Bleeding*: A common symptom is the presence of bright red blood in the stool or on toilet paper after a bowel movement. This is often caused by irritation or friction affecting the internal hemorrhoids.

▸ *Prolapse*: In some cases, internal hemorrhoids may protrude through the anal canal during bowel movements or even while at rest. While they often retract on their own, more severe cases may require medical intervention to reposition them.

▸ *Discomfort*: Many individuals report a sensation of fullness, pressure, or heaviness in the anal area, resulting from the swelling and enlargement of internal hemorrhoids.

▸ **External Hemorrhoids**: External hemorrhoids are located beneath the skin surrounding the anus and are typically more visible and painful than internal hemorrhoids. Positioned below the dentate line, they may be covered by skin or exhibit a purple hue. The most common symptoms include:

▸ *Pain*: External hemorrhoids often cause intense pain, particularly when sitting, walking, or during bowel movements. This discomfort results from the pressure exerted on the swollen veins.

▸ *Itching and Irritation*: The skin surrounding the anus may become irritated, leading to discomfort and itching, due to the constant contact with external hemorrhoids and the associated friction.

▸ *Hemorrhoidal Thrombosis*: In some cases, a blood clot may develop within an external hemorrhoid, a condition known as hemorrhoidal thrombosis. This causes severe, sharp pain and significant swelling in the affected area.

It is important to note that some people may experience both internal and external hemorrhoids simultaneously. Furthermore, internal hemorrhoids can prolapse and protrude through the anal canal, resulting in mixed hemorrhoids, which combine the characteristics and symptoms of both types.

SUBTYPES OF HEMORRHOIDS

In addition to internal and external hemorrhoids, there are less common subtypes that carry clinical significance. These subtypes are defined by specific characteristics and often require tailored treatment approaches. Below are some examples:

‣ **Prolapsed Hemorrhoids**: These are defined by the displacement or protrusion of internal hemorrhoids through the anal canal, which may occur during bowel movements or even at rest. In some cases, they must be manually repositioned. Prolapsed hemorrhoids can be classified as internal or external. Depending on the extent of the protruded tissue, they may vary in pain levels, ranging from mild discomfort to significant distress.

‣ **Thrombosed Hemorrhoids**: This subtype occurs when a blood clot forms within an external hemorrhoid, leading to pronounced swelling. Thrombosed hemorrhoids cause sharp, severe pain in the affected area. They often present as bluish or purplish lumps near the edge of the anus and commonly require medical treatment to alleviate pain and reduce swelling.

‣ **Mixed Hemorrhoids**: This subtype involves the coexistence of both internal and external hemorrhoids. Mixed hemorrhoids may cause pain and display symptoms characteristic of both types. Successfully managing mixed hemorrhoids typically requires a comprehensive treatment plan that addresses both internal and external components to ensure effective relief.

‣ **Hemorrhoid Grades**: Hemorrhoids are classified into different grades based on their severity, using a scale ranging from I to IV. This classification assists in determining the seriousness of the condition and guiding the appropriate treatment:

‣ *Grade I*: These hemorrhoids are small and remain within

the anal canal without prolapsing. They generally do not cause significant symptoms, though mild bleeding during bowel movements may occasionally occur.

‣ *Grade II*: Hemorrhoids in this grade may protrude from the anal canal during bowel movements but spontaneously return to their position afterward. Symptoms can include bleeding and mild discomfort.

‣ *Grade III*: In this case, hemorrhoids prolapse during bowel movements and do not return to their position on their own. Manual repositioning is necessary to place them back inside the anal canal.

‣ *Grade IV*: These hemorrhoids remain continuously prolapsed and cannot be manually reintroduced into the anal canal. They are often very painful and typically require medical or surgical intervention.

It is important to recognize that the evaluation and management of hemorrhoids should be individualized. If you experience related symptoms, consult a physician for an accurate diagnosis and a treatment plan tailored to your specific needs.

Causes

Hemorrhoids, also known as piles, are swollen and inflamed veins located in the rectal and anal region. While this condition is quite common, its exact causes are not yet fully understood. However, various factors may significantly contribute to their development. The following is a more detailed explanation of the potential causes of hemorrhoids:

MOST COMMON CAUSES

‣ **Excessive pressure on the veins**: The leading cause of hemorrhoids is excessive pressure on the veins in the anal region. This can occur due to several factors, such as chronic constipation, excessive straining during bowel movements, pregnancy and childbirth. Prolonged pressure on the veins hinders blood flow, leading to swelling and dilation of the hemorrhoidal veins.

‣ **Chronic constipation**: Frequent constipation and difficulty passing stool increase pressure on the veins in the anal area. Hard, dry stools require extra effort to pass, which can contribute to developing hemorrhoids. Lack of fiber in the diet, insufficient fluid intake and a sedentary lifestyle may contribute to chronic constipation.

▸ **Pregnancy and childbirth:** During pregnancy, the increased weight of the uterus puts pressure on the veins in the pelvis, which can impede blood flow and lead to hemorrhoids. In addition, straining during childbirth can further aggravate this condition. It is common for hemorrhoids that develop during pregnancy to disappear after delivery, but in some cases, they may persist.

▸ **Chronic diarrhea:** Although hemorrhoids are usually associated with constipation, chronic diarrhea can also be a cause. Frequent, watery diarrhea can irritate anal and rectal veins, which can lead to inflammation and hemorrhoid formation.

▸ **Hereditary factors:** Evidence suggests that you may have a genetic predisposition. If you have a family history of hemorrhoids, you may have an increased risk of developing this condition.

Hemorrhoids are not directly inherited, but the predisposition to develop them may be related to weakness of the connective tissue, which supports other tissues. This weakness can lead to hemorrhoids elongating and protruding through the rectum. In addition, people with this hereditary predisposition may be more prone to developing various hernias and drooping organs such as the kidney, bowel, or female genital organs.

▸ **Sedentary lifestyle:** Spending long periods sitting, especially in an uncomfortable position or on hard surfaces, can increase pressure on the veins in the anal area and contribute to the development of hemorrhoids. In addition, a lack of regular physical activity can affect the circulatory system and increase the risk of hemorrhoids.

▸ **Aging:** As we age, the body's tissues become less elastic and resilient. This loss of elasticity can affect the veins and contribute to the development of hemorrhoids in older people.

▸ **Obesity:** Excess body weight can contribute to the formation or worsening of hemorrhoids due to increased abdominal pressure on the pelvic floor. This additional pressure can put stress on the anal and rectal veins, causing them to swell and dilate.

▸ **Bowel movements:** The way we defecate can be one of the most critical factors in the development of hemorrhoids, both in cases of constipation and diarrhea. There are two possible scenarios:

› *Chronic constipation:* Straining during bowel movements can cause the hemorrhoids to dilate, increasing their tendency to protrude from the rectum. In addition, the passage of hard stool can irritate the hemorrhoids, further aggravating the condition.

› *Chronic diarrhea:* Although they do not usually cause hemorrhoids directly, they can trigger a hemorrhoidal crisis. In these cases, the stool is usually more irritating to both the hemorrhoids and the anus, which can result in ruptured blood vessels or intense and uncomfortable irritation.

› **Existence of circulatory disorders or varicose veins:** Circulatory disorders and varicose veins may contribute to the development of hemorrhoids. These conditions affect blood flow and proper circulation in the anal and rectal area, increasing the risk of inflammation and dilation of the hemorrhoidal veins.

DIETARY CAUSES

Some factors of an inadequate diet can influence the development of hemorrhoids, as they can cause dilation of the veins and trigger hemorrhoidal crises due to their abuse. They are the following:

› **Excessive alcohol consumption:** The higher the alcohol content in beverages, the greater the dilatation of hemorrhoids may be.

› **Spicy foods:** These foods can dilate veins, including hemorrhoids.

› **Coffee:** Coffee is usually acceptable in small quantities, but can dilate the veins in high quantities.

› **Seafood:** The abuse of seafood can cause a hemorrhoidal crisis.

› **Excess of acidic foods:** Excessive consumption of citrus fruits such as oranges, lemons, pineapples, strawberries, and grapefruit, as well as acids such as vinegar, can cause the stool to be acidic and, when expelled, irritate the hemorrhoids and the skin of the anus. This is more evident in people who suffer from anal fissures or who have wounds due to previous surgeries in the anorectal area.

‣ **Salted foods**: Very salty foods, such as herring, strong cheeses, olives, and anchovies, can cause fluid retention and hemorrhoids to swell.

‣ **Chocolate**: Cocoa tends to cause constipation, a predisposing factor for hemorrhoidal crises.

FEMALE HORMONES

‣ **Pregnancy**: During pregnancy, the body secretes hormones that increase the diameter of blood vessels, allowing greater blood flow. This predisposes to the appearance of hemorrhoids and varicose veins. In addition, from the sixth month, the baby can exert pressure on the blood vessels, which can cause rupture of the veins surrounding the anus, leading to thrombosis or hematoma. All this, added to constipation that often accompanies pregnancy, worsens the condition of hemorrhoids.

‣ **Childbirth**: Childbirth can worsen hemorrhoids. The hours of dilation, the use of enemas, having a large baby, the passage of the baby through the vaginal canal, the use of forceps and the expulsion of hard stool retained during delivery, all these factors can trigger hemorrhoidal crises, usually intense.

‣ **Menstruation**: During these days, the possibility of experiencing hemorrhoidal crises increases, especially during the "premenstrual syndrome". These crises can manifest themselves in different degrees:

> ‣ Inflammation of the anus or congestive anitis (red anitis): There is swelling and irritation with redness and, in some cases, slight blood loss.

> ‣ Bluish swelling of the anal area with a tendency to protrusion of the hemorrhoids outwards (blue anitis).

> ‣ Thrombosis or perianal hematomas (purple anitis): Blood vessels are ruptured, resulting in clot formation and swelling.

> ‣ Swelling of the skin and folds at the edge of the anus, known as "perianal skin tags".

UNDERLYING DISEASE

At other times, dilated hemorrhoidal veins may be a symptom of an underlying general disease.

‣ **Portal hypertension**: This refers to increased venous pressure in the portal system, which can cause dilation of the hemorrhoidal veins.

Hemorrhoids sometimes occur when blood from the hemorrhoidal veins encounters obstacles in its recirculation through the liver. This can happen in **cirrhosis**, a liver disease that reduces liver function and hinders blood circulation within the liver. Other diseases where hemorrhoids may appear are **hydatidosis**, a disease caused by parasites.

MEDICINES

Certain medicines, such as the following, can also cause hemorrhoids:

‣ **Medications administered rectally**: Suppositories to reduce fever, antirheumatics, etc. These medications can cause both internal and external irritation.

‣ **Medications administered orally**: Acetylsalicylic acid (aspirin), some anti-influenza drugs, contraceptive pills, and certain medicines against arteriosclerosis often cause hemorrhoidal crises. In addition, aspirin, an anticoagulant, can increase the frequency and difficulty of stopping rectal bleeding and relax the connective tissue of hemorrhoids, facilitating their protrusion.

‣ **Anticoagulants**: Their detrimental effect is more significant if bleeding hemorrhoids occur.

‣ **Products for the skin near the anus**: Some soaps, gels, creams or ointments may cause allergic reactions or irritation in some people, which may result in dermatitis or inflammation of the skin of the anus (anodermitis) or inflammation inside the rectum (rectitis).

‣ **Laxatives**: They can be harmful if they cause persistent diarrhea or are taken for long periods, as they irritate the anal area. Some laxatives, such as castor oil, cascara sagrada, rhubarb and aloe vera (when containing aloin), can cause significant irritation. Those containing picosulfate or bisacodyl can also irritate.

▸ **Enemas or enemas:** Some enemas may irritate. To avoid irritation or burning of the rectal mucosa, it is recommended not to use them at very cold or hot temperatures. If salt, pepper, or soap is used in a homemade enema, mixing a maximum of 3 teaspoons of baking soda per liter of water is advisable.

▸ **Vasodilators:** Some cerebral vasodilators, which dilate blood vessels in the brain, can also dilate hemorrhoids.

▸ **Barium pellets** are used in some radiological tests as a contrast. In many cases, after their use, tough stools are formed that are difficult to expel, which can sometimes cause an anal fissure requiring surgery. To avoid this, it is advisable to take a laxative simultaneously.

PHYSICAL STRUCTURE

Tall, thin people are more likely to experience protrusion of their internal hemorrhoids out of the anus. On the other hand, short, stocky, and robust people tend to have internal hemorrhoids that become engorged and enlarged and are more prone to bleeding. If, in addition, a tall person spends all day standing or a stout person works sitting down, this tendency is even more accentuated.

TYPE OF WORK

Those who spend most of the day sitting or standing, predominantly statically, are more prone to hemorrhoidal crises, especially if they have weak connective tissue. Even walking long distances when hemorrhoids are already outside the anus is not recommended.

SOME SPORTS

Certain sports can influence the appearance of hemorrhoids, such as mountaineering (due to the pressure of heights), weightlifting (due to the effort in squatting), cycling (especially in people prone to or with varicose veins or poor circulation in the legs), rowing (due to the effort made with open legs), motocross (due to violent blows in the anal area) and rally driving (due to spending many hours behind the wheel, emotional stress, eating dry and salty foods and drinking a lot of coffee).

SEXUAL LIFE

It is not that sexual activity causes hemorrhoids, but those who already have external hemorrhoids may experience discomfort during or after intercourse due to blood congestion in the pelvic area. In addition, the pain caused by thrombosis makes sexual intercourse almost impossible.

OTHER TRIGGERING CIRCUMSTANCES

Bleeding, hemorrhoidal crises and even thrombosis usually occur after excessive exertion, such as an abundant meal with spicy food or seafood, excessive consumption of alcoholic beverages and coffee, heavy lifting with great effort, episodes of intense diarrhea, or after a long car trip with little rest and poor nutrition.

Possible Complications

This section is here to guide you, helping you understand these potential risks with clarity and confidence. By staying informed, you'll feel more empowered to take proactive steps to safeguard your well-being and prevent these complications from affecting your daily life.

While hemorrhoids are generally a benign condition, in some cases, they can lead to complications of varying severity, which may require medical attention. These complications can significantly impact the quality of life and overall well-being of those affected. Below is a list of the most common complications associated with hemorrhoids:

▸ **Hemorrhoidal thrombosis**: This is the most frequent complication and occurs when a blood clot forms in a hemorrhoid. It is characterized by severe, sharp pain in the affected area. Hemorrhoidal thrombosis can cause the hemorrhoid to become very tender to the touch and can cause significant swelling. Sometimes, it may require surgical drainage to relieve pain and swelling. It can occur in both external and internal hemorrhoids.

▸ *External thrombosis*: It is common to experience pain during defecation that gradually increases and is localized in a specific place at the edge of the anus. It usually occurs after consuming alcohol in excess, eating large amounts of seafood or spicy foods, or during episodes of diarrhea or constipation. The intense pain usually lasts 2 to 3 days, then gradually decreases and usually disappears after 1 to 2 weeks.

In most cases, it heals spontaneously, but in some cases, it may require surgical removal without hospitalization. Occasionally, a fold of skin or "hemorrhoidal shellfish" may remain; in other cases, it leaves no trace. It is also possible to experience several hemorrhoidal thromboses on successive days.

‣ *Internal thrombosis*: In some cases, complications that occur in external hemorrhoids can also occur in internal hemorrhoids, but the pain may be mild or nonexistent and can only be detected during a medical examination. At other times, one of the most painful complications may occur: hemorrhoidal strangulation, which occurs when hemorrhoids tend to protrude, and the anal sphincter squeezes them. The pain is very intense and can extend to the perineum and pelvis. The pain is more intense after bowel movements and can make it difficult to walk and even affect urinary output. This pain may last up to 10 days, so in this case, surgery is recommended as soon as possible. If strangulation occurs, it is crucial to see your doctor immediately, as the problems that can result from this complication could be severe.

If you are facing a thrombosis and do not wish to undergo surgery or must wait for the intervention, it is recommended to follow these tips:

‣ Complete bed rest, elevating the pelvis with a pillow.

‣ Follow the "Foods and Beverages to Avoid During Hemorrhoidal Crisis" recommendations in this book's "Foods That Transform" chapter.

‣ Correct diarrhea or constipation. Ideally, stools should be soft in consistency.

‣ Take venous tonics in high doses. See the "Medicinal Plants" chapter in this book for available options.

‣ You can perform warm or cold sitz baths or use ice cubes in water. Never apply ice directly to the area, which may cause necrosis or tissue death.

‣ Apply a corticosteroid ointment to reduce inflammation.

‣ Gently massage the area with a heparinoid ointment twice or thrice daily.

‣ **Anemia:** Chronic hemorrhoids can cause enough blood loss to cause anemia and decrease red blood cells. This condition can cause weakness, fatigue, pallor, and shortness of breath. To prevent anemia, it is crucial to treat and control bleeding hemorrhoids.

‣ **Hemorrhoidal strangulation:** This occurs when the internal hemorrhoids protrude, and the anal sphincter strangles them, causing blood to stagnate and clot. This results in considerable swelling and makes it difficult or impossible to reintroduce them. This complication is very painful; the pain is constant and can be desperate. In addition, if not appropriately treated, serious complications can arise, such as severe necrosis, local and generalized infection, possible bleeding, and pain, causing insomnia and even shock.

If you experience hemorrhoidal strangulation, it is crucial to see a medical specialist. In situations of isolation or when medical attention is not immediately accessible, the following advice can be followed:

‣ Complete bed rest, elevating the pelvis with a pillow.

‣ Follow the "Foods and Beverages to Avoid During Hemorrhoidal Crisis" recommendations.

‣ Correct diarrhea or constipation to achieve stools of a pasty consistency, avoiding hard or liquid stools.

‣ Take venous tonics in high doses.

‣ Take warm or cold sitz baths or baths with ice cubes in the water, avoiding applying ice directly to the area.

‣ If you experience constipation, take a mild laxative or make a small enema with a rubber bulb and 50 cc of slightly warm olive oil, holding it for about 5 minutes.

‣ If swelling is severe, take a mild diuretic and consume salt-free foods to decrease swelling by increasing the frequency of urination.

‣ In case of severe pain, take an analgesic.

‣ If the hemorrhoids are externalized, lie on your back in bed, relax, apply an ointment, and try to reintroduce them carefully. If this is unsuccessful, it is crucial to see a specialist.

It is still possible to reintroduce them within two hours of their exit. Waiting longer makes the reintroduction process very difficult and even impossible.

‣ In many cases, the most effective solution is surgical intervention.

‣ **Hemorrhoidal crisis:** Anal and rectal discomfort is present, with a sensation of heaviness and a desire to defecate, but no continuous sharp pain is experienced; occasional, short-lasting pinching is experienced. The swelling may affect the entire anal orifice or only some areas, but they do not become hard as in the case of thrombosis, and the pain is not as intense or localized. Although it is not necessary to undergo surgery, many people decide to do so because of the recurrence of the attacks.

If you are in the middle of a hemorrhoidal crisis and do not wish to undergo surgery or must wait for an intervention, complete bed rest is recommended, elevating the pelvis with a pillow. It is also essential to follow the recommendations on foods to avoid in case of a hemorrhoidal crisis and correct any diarrhea or constipation problem to achieve pasty stools, avoiding hard or liquid stools. In addition, it is suggested that tonics be taken in high doses and warm or cold sitz baths or ice cubes in water, always avoiding direct contact with the ice in the affected area. Suppositories or ointments can also be used.

In general, hemorrhoidal crises tend to improve and even disappear with changes in the weather, decreased menstrual flow, and after a few days of controlling food and fluid intake.

‣ **Anal fissure:** This is a chronic tear in the skin of the anus. When ulcerated, they reach the muscle where the sensitive nerve is located, causing intense pain. This condition can occur in young people with few or no hemorrhoids and is considered a true anal fissure. Occasionally, ulceration occurs over a hemorrhoid, causing more bleeding than in the case of a true fissure since the lesion is located over a pocket of blood, which is the hemorrhoid.

The pain caused by a fissure is one of the most intense that can be experienced. It originates during defecation, with a tearing sensation accompanied by slight bleeding in some cases. After 10 to 15 minutes, anal pain begins and increases in intensity until it becomes almost unbearable. This pain usually does not go away with analgesics and may last for several hours, approximately 6 to 8 hours. It then disappears and returns the next day under the same circumstances. This characteristic pain only occurs in two other conditions: anal neuralgia and cryptopapillitis.

Diagnosis of a fissure is simple because it causes characteristic pain and is easily visible on inspection. Slight bleeding may stain the stool laterally, like a streak. A fissure can become infected, causing an abscess, opening, and leaving a fistula.

Suppose you are facing a fissure and must wait for surgery. In that case, it is recommended to follow the recommendations on foods to avoid in case of hemorrhoidal crisis and correct any diarrhea or constipation. In addition, warm or hot sitz baths are suggested, but it is essential to dry the area well with a cool air dryer. You can also apply an ointment with an anesthetic effect to relieve pain and take some analgesics. If the pain does not disappear at any time of the day or night and becomes throbbing, accompanied by fever, this indicates that an abscess is forming under the fissure, so you should see a medical specialist.

▶ **Papillitis and cryptitis:** Morgagni's crypts are small holes inside the anal canal that become inflamed, causing symptoms similar to an anal fissure. This includes intense pain after defecation that disappears after a few hours and recurs under the same circumstances. However, the pain is less intense and of shorter duration compared to an anal fissure. These inflammations can also lead to the formation of fistulas or ulcers, which are usually more extensive than fissures. The causes of these inflammations may include diarrhea, constipation, certain medications, intestinal parasites, urinary and gynecological infections, and the use of some laxatives and enemas.

▶ **Discomfort in the prostate area:** Internal hemorrhoids can cause pain that is felt in the prostate area due to the proximity between the two regions.

▶ **Difficulty urinating:** After hemorrhoid surgery or in cases of anal fissure, there may be difficulty urinating because the pain causes a contraction of the urethral sphincter, preventing the typical passage of urine.

▶ **Persistent bleeding:** It is crucial to keep in mind that not all rectal bleeding is caused by hemorrhoids, so it is essential to have your doctor make the proper diagnosis. If you have already been diagnosed with hemorrhoids and are experiencing light bleeding, you can take the following measures: complete bed rest and elevate your pelvis with a pillow. In addition, it is essential to follow the recommendations on foods to avoid in case of a hemorrhoidal crisis and to correct any diarrhea or constipation problems. You can also take a venotonic preparation to help control bleeding.

However, if the bleeding persists and lasts more than a day, you must see your doctor for further evaluation. If the bleeding is severe, seeking emergency medical attention at the nearest medical center is necessary.

▸ **Infection**: In some cases, hemorrhoids can become infected, causing pain, swelling, and redness in the affected area. Infection can occur if the hemorrhoids are injured or ruptured due to friction or excessive scratching. If infection is suspected, seek medical attention for antibiotic treatment.

▸ **Hemorrhoid prolapse**: In more severe cases, hemorrhoids can prolapse or slip out of the anus. This occurs when the internal hemorrhoids slide out of the anus. Hemorrhoid prolapse can cause pain, discomfort and difficulty with bowel movements. In some cases, prolapse may require medical or surgical treatment to return the hemorrhoids to their normal position.

▸ **Chronic constipation**: Hemorrhoids can make constipation worse, and in turn, constipation can make hemorrhoids worse. Difficulty passing stool can increase pressure on the veins in the anal and rectal region, which can aggravate existing hemorrhoids or cause new hemorrhoids to develop. Maintaining a balanced diet, drinking enough water, and engaging in regular physical activity are essential to prevent constipation.

▸ **Severe bleeding**: In rare cases, hemorrhoids may bleed very heavily and persistently, which may require emergency medical attention. Severe bleeding can cause anemia and extreme weakness and may require blood transfusions or surgery to stop the bleeding.

▸ **Hemorrhoidal ulcer**: In severe hemorrhoids, constant pressure and inflammation can cause ulcers in the hemorrhoid tissue. These ulcers can be painful and take longer to heal than ordinary hemorrhoids. Proper treatment and symptom management are necessary to promote the healing of ulcers.

▸ **Anal fistulas**: Chronic hemorrhoids can cause anal fistulas to form. An anal fistula is an abnormal passage that forms between the anal canal and the skin near the anus. This can result in pain, swelling and persistent discharge. Anal fistulas usually require surgical intervention for treatment.

‣ **Fecal incontinence**: In sporadic and severe cases, advanced and untreated hemorrhoids can contribute to the development of fecal incontinence. This is because hemorrhoids can damage the muscles and nerves of the anal sphincter, which can lead to the inability to control bowel movements. Fecal incontinence can have a significant impact on quality of life and may require specialized medical treatment.

It is important to note that not everyone with hemorrhoids will experience these complications. Most hemorrhoids can be effectively treated and managed with lifestyle changes, topical treatments and other non-invasive treatments. However, if you experience severe symptoms or complications, seeking medical attention for proper diagnosis and treatment is critical.

In addition, it is essential to maintain good anal hygiene, avoid constipation through a diet rich in fiber and fluids, exercise regularly and avoid excessive straining during bowel movements. It is always advisable to consult a physician if you have any concerns or if symptoms persist.

Symptoms Reduction and Prevention

Reducing symptoms and preventing the development of hemorrhoids are crucial for enhancing quality of life and avoiding potential complications. Incorporating healthy habits and adhering to specific recommendations can have a significant impact on effectively managing this condition. The following outlines practical steps and useful tips to help achieve this:

‣ **Maintain good anal hygiene**: It is important to gently clean the anal area after each bowel movement. It is recommended to use soft toilet paper or alcohol-free wipes. Avoid excessive rubbing or scratching, as this can irritate hemorrhoids.

‣ **Avoid constipation**: Constipation is one of the primary triggers of hemorrhoids. To prevent it, follow a fiber-rich diet and consume fruits, vegetables, whole grains, and legumes. In addition, drink enough water to maintain adequate hydration and facilitate intestinal transit.

‣ **Avoid excessive straining during defecation**: It is essential to avoid prolonged and excessive straining during bowel movements, as this can increase pressure on the veins in the anal area. A stool can elevate the legs and adopt a more suitable position to facilitate evacuation if necessary.

▸ **Maintain a healthy weight**: Being overweight and obese can increase pressure on the veins in the anal area, which increases the risk of developing hemorrhoids. Maintaining a healthy weight through a balanced diet and regular exercise can help prevent the appearance of.

▸ **Avoid a sedentary** lifestyle: A sedentary lifestyle can contribute to the development of hemorrhoids. Regular physical activity, such as walking, swimming, or yoga, improves blood circulation and prevents hemorrhoids.

▸ **Do not sit or stand for long periods**: Both sitting for many hours at a time and standing for long periods can put pressure on the veins in the anal area. Getting up and moving around occasionally is recommended, primarily if you work in a static position.

▸ **Avoid excessive use of laxatives**: Prolonged and excessive use of laxatives can weaken bowel muscles and worsen constipation in the long run. It is essential to use laxatives only when necessary and under the supervision of a physician.

▸ **Do not postpone the urge to defecate**: Withholding the urge to defecate for too long can lead to hardening of the stool and make bowel movements more difficult. Attending to the need to defecate as soon as possible is essential.

▸ **Avoid excessive use of irritating products**: Some personal hygiene products, such as perfumed soaps, can irritate and worsen hemorrhoid symptoms. It is essential to use mild, hypoallergenic products to care for the anal area.

▸ **Avoid excessive consumption of alcohol and spices**: Alcohol and spicy foods can irritate the lining of the bowel and increase the inflammation of hemorrhoids. Limiting their consumption may help reduce symptoms.

▸ **Sitz baths**: Sitz baths with warm water can relieve and reduce the inflammation of hemorrhoids. Soaking the anal area in warm water for 10-15 minutes several times a day is recommended. Ingredients such as Epsom salt or baking soda can also be added to the water for relief.

‣ **Apply hot or cold compresses**: Applying hot or cold compresses to the affected area can help reduce swelling and relieve discomfort. Cold compresses, wrapped in a cloth and filled with ice, or hot compresses, soaked in warm water, can be used. Alternating between hot and cold compresses may provide further relief.

‣ **Avoid excessive use of painkillers**: Excessive use of painkillers such as ibuprofen or acetaminophen can worsen hemorrhoid symptoms, as they can cause constipation. It is essential to use these drugs only when necessary and under the supervision of a physician.

‣ **Avoid tobacco use**: Smoking can worsen hemorrhoid symptoms by compromising blood circulation and increasing inflammation. Quitting or reducing tobacco use can help relieve symptoms and improve overall health.

‣ **Maintain proper weight control during pregnancy**: During pregnancy, hemorrhoids are common due to increased pressure on the veins in the anal area. Maintaining proper weight control, eating a balanced diet, and exercising under the supervision of a physician can help prevent or control hemorrhoids during pregnancy.

‣ **Avoid heavy lifting**: Lifting heavy objects can increase pressure on the veins in the anal area and worsen hemorrhoid symptoms. It is essential to avoid heavy lifting and, if necessary, use proper lifting techniques to reduce the strain on the affected area.

Additional Recommendations

Proper management of hemorrhoids often involves adopting specific practices that complement basic preventive measures. These additional recommendations can help alleviate discomfort, prevent irritation, and support a faster recovery. Outlined below are practical, easy-to-follow tips for addressing particular situations, such as repositioning external hemorrhoids, maintaining optimal stool care, and utilizing natural remedies to relieve symptoms and prevent constipation.

‣ **If hemorrhoids come out during defecation**, it is advisable to carefully reintroduce them. This can be done by lying on your back, bending the legs, relaxing, and gently pushing them back with clean fingers. Another option is sitting on a towel at the edge of the bathtub for better support. Always ensure the process is done calmly and without applying excessive force.

‣ **When hemorrhoids remain outside and cannot be reintroduced**, it is essential to protect them from irritation. Friction caused by rubbing against underwear can worsen discomfort, so it's best to avoid wearing tight-fitting clothing. Opt for loose, breathable fabrics that minimize contact with the sensitive area and help reduce inflammation.

‣ **Maintaining soft bowel movements** is another key aspect of managing this condition. Stools should be soft to avoid exacerbating the problem, but they should not be too liquid, as this might irritate the hemorrhoids further. If constipation or tough stools are an issue, addressing them promptly is important. Otherwise, the internal hemorrhoids may struggle to heal.

‣ **As a quick remedy**, a stool softener can be used for a few days, under the guidance of a pharmacist or doctor. However, for long-term relief, it's necessary to address the root cause, especially if constipation tends to recur frequently. Taking proactive steps can greatly improve daily comfort and prevent further complications.

‣ **For long-term management**, natural remedies can help regulate bowel movements. If you tend to suffer from constipation or have very dry and hard stools, try soaking a tablespoon of psyllium, flax, or linseed in a glass of water for a few hours. In the evening, drink the entire contents, including the seeds, slightly warmed. Another natural option is to drink warm water with honey first thing in the morning on an empty stomach. Coconut oil, consumed before breakfast and dinner, may also provide gentle relief. These remedies can help maintain regularity and support healing over time.

Local Hygiene

Maintaining proper local hygiene is crucial for minimizing discomfort caused by hemorrhoids and preventing additional infections or irritation. Thorough and gentle care of the area, particularly after bowel movements, can significantly enhance symptom relief and promote overall recovery. Below are practical and careful guidelines for cleansing and drying the affected area to ensure comfort and prevent complications.

‣ **Wash Instead of Wiping**: When hemorrhoids protrude, it is better to wash the area with water instead of wiping with toilet paper, as wiping can cause further irritation. For internal hemorrhoids, gentle wiping with soft toilet paper is generally acceptable.

▸ **Water Temperature Matters**: Always use cool or slightly warm water for washing. Avoid hot water, as it can dilate the blood vessels, aggravating hemorrhoids and increasing the risk of bleeding.

▸ **After Bowel Movements**: Wash the area with warm or cool water after every bowel movement. Dry toilet paper can irritate the sensitive mucous membrane, potentially worsening symptoms or trapping fecal matter in the hemorrhoid, leading to further complications. After washing, gently pat the area dry using a soft towel or absorbent material, avoiding any rubbing.

▸ **Use of Wet Wipes**: Wet wipes specifically designed for sensitive areas can be a good alternative. Always use wipes with gentle touches to avoid aggravating the condition. If you're away from home, you can moisten wet wipes, gauze, or cotton pads to clean yourself. Allow the area to air-dry completely to prevent moisture, which can lead to skin irritation.

▸ **Sitz Baths for Relief**: During hemorrhoidal flare-ups, a sitz bath with cool water or even ice-cold water can provide relief. This can be done for 2 to 3 days but should not become a daily routine. Avoid placing ice cubes directly on the skin. Instead, wrap them in a thin cloth or gauze to prevent tissue damage or necrosis. Keep sitz baths brief to avoid over-softening the skin.

▸ **Soap Use**: If you choose to use soap, opt for neutral or hypoallergenic formulas to minimize skin irritation.

▸ **Drying the Area**: After washing and patting the area dry, you can use a hairdryer on a cool (non-hot) setting for 1-2 minutes to ensure the skin is completely dry without causing further irritation.

Everyday Care

Effectively managing hemorrhoids involves cultivating gentle habits and implementing mindful lifestyle changes. From hygiene practices to dietary adjustments, these strategies can help reduce discomfort, prevent additional complications, and promote a smoother recovery. Below is a comprehensive guide to everyday care:

‣ **Hygiene:** To avoid injury and reduce the risk of infection, never scratch or rub hemorrhoids. Be gentle during hygiene routines, and if bathing, prefer showers over baths. This helps prevent skin softening. Use cold or lukewarm water, and keep hot showers brief to minimize irritation.

‣ **Extreme Heat:** Extreme heat can be harmful in certain circumstances. Sweltering saunas, for example, can exacerbate issues if hemorrhoids are exposed. However, if they do not protrude, short sauna sessions are acceptable, provided they are interspersed with cold showers to stimulate circulation.

‣ **Exercise:** Exercise plays a vital role in hemorrhoid care, with walking being particularly beneficial as it facilitates bowel movements and mitigates constipation–one of the primary causes of hemorrhoids. However, avoid exercises involving heavy lifting or open-legged movements as they can worsen symptoms.

‣ **Toilet Posture:** When using the toilet, reduce defecation time, limiting it to no more than 10 minutes. For better posture during defecation, adopt a squatting position or place your feet on a stool approximately 20 cm high. This posture reduces strain and helps prevent hemorrhoids from protruding.

‣ **Diet and Digestive Care:** Maintaining healthy dietary habits is essential, especially during a "hemorrhoidal crisis". To reduce symptoms, avoid irritating foods like excessively spicy or greasy dishes, alcohol, and even decaffeinated coffee. Instead, prioritize a fiber-rich diet that includes fruits, vegetables, whole grains, and wheat bran, which supports optimal digestion and regular bowel movements. Ensure you drink around 2 liters of water daily to prevent constipation and promote softer stools. Achieving a stool consistency that is soft but not liquid is crucial to minimize discomfort and bleeding, making it important to adjust your diet and hydration to strike this balance effectively.

‣ **Pelvic Strength:** Regularly practicing anal and Kegel exercises can significantly improve symptoms, enhance circulation, and strengthen the muscles around the anus. To perform them, contract the anal sphincter inward as if holding back feces while simultaneously engaging the pelvic floor muscles by squeezing and lifting them upward. These exercises, when done daily, not only alleviate discomfort but also help prevent future hemorrhoidal issues.

▸ **Seating**: When choosing seating, avoid excessively rigid surfaces or materials that block air circulation, such as plastic, wood, or iron. Similarly, seats that sink too deeply should be avoided.

▸ **Clothing**: For clothing, ensure it is loose and breathable, especially if hemorrhoids protrude externally. Avoid tight-fitting garments, thong-style underwear, or anything that causes chafing or inadequate air circulation.

Medication Guidelines

Using medications appropriately is crucial during hemorrhoidal crises, and self-medication should be avoided. Always seek advice from a doctor, pharmacist, or healthcare professional to ensure the treatment is customized to your specific condition. Below are the key considerations for various types of medications:

▸ **Venotonics**: Venotonics, including remedies derived from medicinal plants, can promote healing and reduce symptoms during acute hemorrhoidal episodes. These substances enhance vein function and resilience, accelerating recovery. For detailed insights into the most effective options, refer to the chapter titled Medicinal Plants.

▸ **Topical Ointments**: Topical ointments can offer relief by reducing itching and inflammation. While useful for temporary comfort during flare-ups, they do not address the root cause of the condition. Prolonged or frequent use is discouraged, as it may lead to side effects like anal dermatitis or skin atrophy.

▸ **Vasoconstrictor Creams**: Creams with vasoconstrictor properties should be used cautiously, especially for individuals with hypertension. These products can constrict blood vessels, potentially worsening cardiovascular health. If you have high blood pressure, consult your doctor or pharmacist for safer alternatives that will effectively manage symptoms without compromising heart health.

▸ **Vitamin C and Flavonoids**: Vitamin C and flavonoids are beneficial for vein health, boosting vascular resilience and reducing inflammation. Incorporating these nutrients into your diet or exploring suitable supplements under medical guidance can complement your hemorrhoidal treatment.

▶ **Special Considerations for Diabetes**: People with diabetes must avoid creams or ointments containing hydrocortisone, as these can elevate blood sugar levels. Additionally, medications with vasoconstrictors, such as phenylephrine, should be avoided due to their potential impacts on blood sugar management. Speak with your healthcare provider to identify safe and effective treatment options tailored to diabetes-specific needs.

By following these guidelines and consulting professionals, you can ensure safe and effective relief from hemorrhoidal symptoms while minimizing potential risks associated with medication use.

Diagnostic Medical Tests

Diagnostic medical tests are essential in the evaluation and diagnosis of hemorrhoids. They allow for an assessment of their severity and the detection of potential complications. Listed below are the most commonly performed tests:

▶ **Physical exam and review of symptoms**: The doctor will begin with a physical exam of the anal and rectal area, looking for visible signs of external or internal hemorrhoids. They will also review the symptoms you are experiencing, such as itching, pain, bleeding, or lumps.

▶ **Anoscopy**: This test involves an anoscope, a thin, hollow tube with a light. The physician gently inserts it into the anal canal to examine the lower rectum and internal hemorrhoids. Anoscopy allows direct visualization of the hemorrhoids and helps determine their location, size and degree of inflammation

▶ **Proctoscopy**: Similar to anoscopy, proctoscopy uses a proctoscope to examine the lower rectum and internal hemorrhoids. However, unlike anoscopy, the proctoscope is longer and allows for a deeper visualization of the rectum.

▶ **Flexible Rectoscopy**: This test involves inserting a thin, flexible tube called a rectoscope into the rectum to examine the lower rectum and the sigmoid colon. The rectoscope evaluates internal hemorrhoids and can also help rule out other diseases of the rectum and colon.

▶ **Colonoscopy**: A colonoscopy may be performed if other rectal conditions are suspected or a more complete colon evaluation is required. This test uses a colonoscope, a long, flexible tube with a camera on the end, to examine the entire colon for abnormalities, including hemorrhoids.

▸ **Imaging tests:** In rare cases where a severe complication of hemorrhoids, such as a thrombus or anal fissure, is suspected, imaging tests, such as ultrasound or MRI, may be used to obtain detailed images of the affected area and determine the extent of the lesion.

▸ **Anorectal manometry:** This test is performed to evaluate the muscular function of the rectum and anal sphincter. A thin catheter is inserted into the rectum, measuring pressure and muscle activity during bowel movements. Anorectal manometry can help identify motility problems or sphincter dysfunctions that may contribute to hemorrhoidal symptoms.

▸ **Defecography:** This test is used to evaluate the function of the rectum and anus during evacuation. It consists of administering a contrast medium through the rectum, followed by X-rays while the person strains to evacuate. Defecography may reveal structural or functional problems that may be related to hemorrhoidal symptoms.

▸ **Sigmoidoscopy:** Similar to colonoscopy, sigmoidoscopy uses a thin, flexible tube called a sigmoidoscope to examine the lining of the sigmoid colon. This test focuses on a specific part of the colon and can help evaluate hemorrhoids in this area.

▸ **Cytology and biopsy:** If a lesion or abnormal mass is suspected, in rare cases, cytology or biopsy may be performed in the rectal area. These tests involve taking a sample of tissue or cells from the affected area for laboratory analysis. Cytology and biopsy can help rule out other, more severe conditions, such as cancer.

It's important to understand that not all the tests mentioned will be necessary in your case. Your doctor will decide which ones are most appropriate based on your symptoms, medical history, and the severity of your hemorrhoids. The goal is to perform only the necessary tests to achieve an accurate diagnosis.

Warning Signs

It is crucial to pay attention to certain symptoms that may indicate a worsening condition or complications related to hemorrhoids. If you experience any of the following signs, consult your doctor immediately or visit an emergency room:

▸ **Abnormal Bleeding:**
  - Anal bleeding that occurs without the need to defecate.
  - Persistent bleeding after bowel movements, even in small amounts.

▸ **Prolonged or Recurrent Pain:**
  - Intense pain that does not subside or continues to worsen over time.
  - Pain or discomfort accompanied by bleeding that lasts for more than a week.

▸ **Changes in Symptoms:**
  - Bleeding that changes in color, shifting from bright red (fresh blood) to dark red, which may suggest a more serious complication.
  - Appearance of new symptoms, such as increased swelling, unusual discharge, or hardening in the anal area.

▸ **Lack of Improvement with Basic Treatments**
  - Despite using home remedies (like sitz baths), improving your diet (e.g., adding more fiber), and staying active, symptoms persist or worsen.

▸ **Severe Associated Symptoms:**
  - Heavy bleeding accompanied by abdominal pain, high fever, or an overall feeling of malaise.
  - Blood mixed with stool, or very dark-colored stools (melena), which may indicate an issue beyond hemorrhoids, such as bleeding elsewhere in the digestive tract.

What to Do If You Notice These Signs

If you experience any of these symptoms, do not ignore them. Prompt medical attention can help prevent serious complications and ensure appropriate treatment. While hemorrhoids are common and treatable, serious warning signs should always be addressed immediately.

FREQUENTLY ASKED QUESTIONS

Navigating the intricate world of health can feel overwhelming, especially when faced with a diagnosis that affects both physical and emotional well-being. In such moments, many questions naturally arise: What does this mean for me? What options are available? How will my daily life change? Uncertainty and concern are common. Here, you'll discover practical and direct insights to help you make confident, informed choices.

This chapter was created to offer support and provide clear, straightforward tools to guide you through this journey. In today's era of abundant information, distinguishing reliable knowledge from content that might cause confusion is vital. With this in mind, I've compiled evidence-based guidance to help you navigate uncertainty with greater clarity.

The format of this resource prioritizes accessibility, addressing common concerns faced by individuals and families alike. Each explanation is concise, clear, and aimed at empowering you to make decisions that align with your overall well-being.

While the material here is designed to assist, it is not a substitute for personalized advice from healthcare professionals. Consulting your doctor for guidance tailored to your specific needs remains essential, especially to address challenges unique to your situation.

Through these pages, my goal is to foster calm, confidence, and reassurance so that you can approach your circumstances with strength and resolve. I hope this resource inspires you and provides the valuable tools necessary to manage your health effectively and confidently.

128 FAQs About Hemorrhoids

1. What are hemorrhoids?
Hemorrhoids are swollen veins in the rectum and anus area that can cause pain, itching and bleeding. They are common and can be internal or external.

2. What are the causes?
Causes may include straining during bowel movements, chronic constipation, pregnancy, obesity, a low-fiber diet and a sedentary lifestyle.

3. What are the symptoms?
Common symptoms include rectal bleeding, itching, pain or discomfort in the anal area, swelling and, in some cases, a lump near the anus.

4. How are hemorrhoids diagnosed?
Hemorrhoids are diagnosed by physical examination, which may include a visual inspection of the anus and a digital exam of the rectum. Additional tests such as anoscopy, sigmoidoscopy, or colonoscopy may be required to rule out other conditions.

5. Can external hemorrhoids become internal?
No. External and internal hemorrhoids differ in location and do not merge, although a person can have both types simultaneously.

6. Do internal and external hemorrhoids require different treatments?
Yes, internal and external hemorrhoids may require different treatment approaches. Internal hemorrhoids are usually treated with dietary changes, medications, or procedures such as rubber band ligation, while external hemorrhoids may require topical creams, sitz baths, or, in severe cases, surgery.

7. Is it safe to use over-the-counter treatments?
Many over-the-counter treatments are safe and effective in relieving temporary symptoms, but it is essential to follow instructions and consult a physician if symptoms persist.

8. What dietary changes can help prevent or treat it?
Increasing fiber intake, with plenty of fruits, vegetables, legumes and whole grains, drinking enough water, and avoiding foods that can cause constipation or irritation can help prevent and manage hemorrhoids by facilitating bowel transit and bowel movements. We will discuss this in detail in the corresponding chapter.

9. How does a low-fiber diet affect hemorrhoids?
A diet low in fiber may contribute to constipation, increasing pressure during bowel movements, and the risk of developing or worsening hemorrhoids.

10. What foods should be avoided?
It is advisable to avoid foods that may cause constipation or irritation, such as processed, spicy, high-fat, and low-fiber foods. We will discuss this in the chapter dedicated to food.

11. Can spicy foods make it worse?
Although they do not cause hemorrhoids, spicy foods can irritate the digestive tract and worsen symptoms in some people.

12. Is it necessary to see a doctor?
It is advisable to consult a physician if you experience persistent symptoms, rectal bleeding, severe pain, or if home treatments do not relieve the discomfort to rule out other, more severe conditions.

13. What type of physician treats hemorrhoids?
Proctologists, also known as coloproctologists, are specialists in the treatment of hemorrhoids and other conditions of the rectum and anus.

14. What is a coloproctologist?
A coloproctologist is a physician who specializes in the diagnosis and treatment of disorders of the colon, rectum and anus, including hemorrhoids.

15. Can they disappear on their own?
Minor hemorrhoids may disappear on their own with changes in diet, lifestyle, and the use of home treatments, but more severe hemorrhoids may require medical intervention.

16. What is pelvic congestion syndrome, and what is its relation to hemorrhoids?
Pelvic congestion syndrome is caused by varicose veins in the pelvis, which may be associated with hemorrhoids due to increased venous pressure.

17. How does pregnancy affect them?
Pregnancy may increase the risk of developing hemorrhoids due to the pressure of the growing uterus on the pelvic veins and hormonal changes that affect blood flow and bowel transit.

18. Does pregnancy always cause hemorrhoids?
Not always, but pregnancy increases the risk of developing hemorrhoids due to hormonal changes, increased abdominal pressure, and constipation at this stage.

19. Is it possible to prevent them during pregnancy?

Although the risk of hemorrhoids increases during pregnancy, preventive measures can be taken, such as maintaining a diet rich in fiber, adequate hydration, walking or swimming, and avoiding standing or sitting for long periods.

20. Is it safe to use hemorrhoid creams during pregnancy?

Many topical hemorrhoid creams are safe to use during pregnancy, but it is essential to consult your doctor before using them to make sure they will not affect the pregnancy.

21. Can it disappear after childbirth?

Yes, in many women, hemorrhoids developed during pregnancy or childbirth tend to improve or disappear after giving birth, especially with changes in diet and lifestyle.

22. Is it possible to treat it during lactation?

Yes, hemorrhoids can be treated during lactation with conservative measures and specific treatments that are safe for the baby. It is essential to consult a healthcare professional to choose the appropriate treatment.

23. How do hormonal changes affect them?

Hormonal changes, such as those that occur during pregnancy and menopause, can affect bowel function and venous pressure, increasing the risk of hemorrhoids.

24. How can menopause affect them?

Menopause can influence bowel habits due to hormonal changes and circulatory disorders, which may increase the risk of constipation and hemorrhoids.

25. Can it cause complications?

Although rarely serious, hemorrhoids can lead to complications such as chronic blood loss anemia, prolapse, or hemorrhoidal thrombosis in more severe cases.

26. Can it affect people of all ages?

Yes, hemorrhoids can affect people of any age, including children, although they are more common in adults over 45 years of age. Factors such as constipation or overexertion can cause them in younger people.

27. Is it possible to completely prevent it?

While complete prevention cannot be guaranteed, maintaining a healthy lifestyle with a diet rich in fiber, adequate hydration, and regular exercise can significantly reduce the risk of developing hemorrhoids.

28. What is the role of exercise in its prevention?
Regular exercise helps improve circulation, maintain a healthy weight, and promote bowel regularity, which can reduce the risk of developing hemorrhoids.

29. What exercises are recommended?
Low-impact exercises like walking, swimming, or yoga can improve circulation and reduce hemorrhoid symptoms.

30. Can yoga help prevent or relieve it?
Yoga and other forms of gentle exercise often improve circulation and digestion, helping to prevent constipation and reducing pressure in the anal area, which can prevent or relieve hemorrhoids.

31. How does intense exercise affect hemorrhoids?
Intense exercise, especially activities that increase abdominal pressure, such as weight lifting, may worsen hemorrhoids by increasing pressure in the anal blood vessels.

32. What is the relationship between weightlifting and hemorrhoids?
Lifting weights with improper technique or excessive exertion can increase intra-abdominal pressure and contribute to the development of hemorrhoids.

33. Are there any home remedies to relieve the symptoms of hemorrhoids?
Some home remedies include sitz baths with warm water, wet wipes instead of toilet paper, cold compresses to reduce swelling, aloe vera or witch hazel, and a fiber-rich diet. This book will discuss these in detail.

34. How does a sedentary lifestyle affect hemorrhoids?
A sedentary lifestyle can contribute to constipation and increase pressure on anal veins, which can increase the risk of developing hemorrhoids.

35. How can the type of work affect hemorrhoids?
Jobs that require sitting or standing for long periods often increase the risk of developing hemorrhoids due to the continuous pressure on the anal region.

36. Can hemorrhoids be hereditary?
They are not directly inherited, but a predisposition to factors that contribute to hemorrhoids, such as connective tissue weakness, may be inherited.

37. What role do genetics play in the development of hemorrhoids?

Genetic predisposition may influence the weakness of the venous walls, increasing the risk of developing hemorrhoids, although environmental and lifestyle factors are also significant.

38. Can hemorrhoids be a sign of another medical condition?

Although hemorrhoids are common and usually not severe, rectal bleeding and other similar symptoms can be signs of more serious conditions, such as colorectal cancer, so it is essential to consult a physician for a proper diagnosis.

39. Can hemorrhoids be a sign of cancer?

Hemorrhoids are not a sign of cancer, but similar symptoms, such as rectal bleeding, should be evaluated by a physician to rule out other more severe conditions.

40. How do hemorrhoids affect quality of life?

Hemorrhoids can cause significant discomfort, making daily activities such as sitting, walking, or going to the bathroom difficult, and can negatively impact quality of life if not properly managed.

41. What is the difference between hemorrhoids and anal fissures?

Hemorrhoids are swollen veins in the anus or rectum, while an anal fissure is a small tear in the skin of the anus, which can cause severe pain and bleeding during bowel movements. They have different causes and treatments.

42. Can the use of laxatives help prevent hemorrhoids?

Laxatives may help relieve occasional constipation, but should not be used as a long-term solution. Frequent use may cause dependence and worsen the problem.

43. Is it safe to use laxatives to treat hemorrhoids?

Occasional use of laxatives may be safe, but prolonged use without medical supervision is not recommended, as it can lead to dependence and worsen constipation and hemorrhoids.

44. Are hemorrhoids more common in men or women?

Hemorrhoids affect both genders, although some studies suggest that they may be slightly more common in women, especially during pregnancy.

45. How long do hemorrhoids usually last?

The duration of hemorrhoids varies depending on their severity and treatment. Minor hemorrhoids may resolve in a few days with proper treatment, while more severe hemorrhoids may require weeks or months.

46. Is it possible to have hemorrhoids without pain?
Yes, especially in the case of internal hemorrhoids, which often do not cause pain due to the lack of nerve endings in the rectum. However, they can cause bleeding or prolapse.

47. What is a prolapsed hemorrhoid or hemorrhoidal prolapse?
A hemorrhoidal prolapse occurs when an internal hemorrhoid becomes so enlarged that it protrudes outside the anus, often during straining during bowel movements. It can be painful and usually requires medical treatment.

48. Can stress contribute to hemorrhoids?
Stress is not a direct cause of hemorrhoids, but it can contribute to constipation and unhealthy habits, such as poor diet, which can increase the risk.

49. What role does hydration play in the prevention?
Adequate hydration helps keep stools soft and facilitates their passage, reducing the need for straining during defecation and the risk of developing hemorrhoids.

50. What drinks are recommended?
Drinking enough water is crucial. Natural juices rich in fiber and herbal teas that do not cause dehydration are also beneficial.

51. How does dehydration affect hemorrhoids?
Dehydration can lead to constipation, which increases the risk of developing or worsening hemorrhoids due to straining during bowel movements.

52. How does alcohol consumption affect hemorrhoids?
Excessive alcohol consumption can cause dehydration and constipation, increasing the risk of developing and worsening hemorrhoids due to the additional pressure on the digestive system.

53. Can hemorrhoids cause fever?
Hemorrhoids do not cause fever. However, if a fever is present, it could indicate an infection or a different underlying condition. In this case, it would be essential to seek medical attention.

54. Is it possible for hemorrhoids to become infected?
Although rare, hemorrhoids can become infected, mainly if they are caused by a break or cut in the skin. Signs of infection include severe pain, fever, redness and pus.

55. How can sitting posture affect hemorrhoids?
Sitting for long periods, especially on hard surfaces, can increase pressure in the anal area, exacerbating hemorrhoid symptoms.

56. How do bowel habits affect the risk of hemorrhoids?
Habits such as excessive straining, spending too much time on the toilet, or ignoring the urge to void can increase the risk of developing hemorrhoids.

57. Can prolonged use of the toilet cause hemorrhoids?
Remaining on the toilet for prolonged periods can increase pressure in the rectal veins, which can contribute to the formation of hemorrhoids.

58. What role does posture during defecation play in preventing hemorrhoids?
Adopting a more natural posture when defecating, such as elevating the feet with a stool, can help align the rectum and facilitate the passage of stool, reducing straining and the risk of hemorrhoids.

59. Can hemorrhoids be prevented with fiber supplements?
Fiber supplements can help soften stools and facilitate intestinal transit, reducing straining and, therefore, the risk of developing hemorrhoids, but should be used as a complement to a balanced diet.

60. How does fiber consumption affect hemorrhoids?
A fiber-rich diet can help relieve hemorrhoids by softening the stool and making it easier to pass, reducing straining during defecation.

61. How does being overweight influence hemorrhoids?
Being overweight can increase pressure on the veins of the rectum and anus, increasing the risk of developing hemorrhoids.

62. How can weight loss help hemorrhoids?
Weight loss can reduce abdominal and pelvic pressure, decreasing the risk and severity of hemorrhoids.

63. Are sitz baths effective in relieving hemorrhoids?
Yes, warm sitz baths can temporarily reduce swelling and relieve hemorrhoid pain.

64. How does smoking affect hemorrhoids?
Smoking can affect circulation and vascular health, which may exacerbate hemorrhoids. In addition, smoking may contribute to constipation due to changes in metabolism.

65. Is the use of wet toilet paper beneficial?
Using unscented wipes may be gentler on irritated skin around the anus than dry toilet paper, which can help prevent irritation.

66. Does the consumption of probiotics help in the management of hemorrhoids?
Probiotics can improve intestinal health and help maintain regularity, reducing the risk of constipation and, in turn, hemorrhoids.

67. Is the use of analgesics recommended for hemorrhoid pain?
Over-the-counter analgesics, such as acetaminophen or ibuprofen, may help relieve pain associated with hemorrhoids, but always follow the guidance of a physician, as they may cause adverse effects on the body in the long term.

68. What treatments are available for hemorrhoids?
Treatments include diet and lifestyle changes, topical or oral medications or supplements, non-surgical procedures such as rubber band ligation, and surgery in severe cases.

69. What is a blood clot in a hemorrhoid?
A blood clot in a hemorrhoid is a thrombosed hemorrhoid, which can be painful and require medical attention.

70. What are thrombosed hemorrhoids?
Thrombosed hemorrhoids are external hemorrhoids in which a blood clot has formed, causing a complex and very painful lump around the anus.

71. Does coffee consumption affect hemorrhoids?
Coffee, due to its caffeine content, can dehydrate and potentially contribute to constipation in some people, which could worsen hemorrhoids.

72. How can hemorrhoids be managed in people with inflammatory bowel disease?

Management of hemorrhoids in people with inflammatory bowel disease should be careful and generally focus on treating the underlying condition, improving diet, and considering topical or surgical treatments under medical supervision.

73. How does aging affect hemorrhoids?
Aging can weaken the supporting tissues in the anal area, making hemorrhoids more likely due to minor strains or changes in bowel motility.

74. Can essential oils be used to treat hemorrhoids?
Some essential oils may have anti-inflammatory and soothing properties, but should be used with caution and under the guidance of a professional to avoid irritation.

75. How are hemorrhoids different from anal polyps?
Hemorrhoids are swollen veins, while anal polyps are tissue growths in the lining of the rectum or anus. Polyps may require further evaluation to rule out malignancy.

76. What are hemorrhoidal pads?
Hemorrhoidal pads are normal tissues in the lower rectum that help control the passage of stool. Hemorrhoids occur when these pads become inflamed or enlarged.

77. Can hemorrhoids cause bleeding without pain?
Yes, especially internal hemorrhoids, which can cause painless bleeding during or after bowel movements.

78. Why is it important not to ignore rectal bleeding?
Rectal bleeding can be a symptom of several conditions, including hemorrhoids, anal fissures, or even colorectal cancer, so it is essential to seek medical attention for an accurate diagnosis.

79. Can hemorrhoids cause changes in stool color?
Hemorrhoids do not change the color of the stool, although bleeding may cause bright red blood spots on the stool or toilet paper.

80. Can hemorrhoids cause anemia?
In cases of chronic bleeding due to hemorrhoids, it is possible to develop iron deficiency anemia, although this is rare.

81. Can hemorrhoids change size over time?
Yes, hemorrhoids can change in size depending on factors such as diet, level of physical activity, and bowel habits. They can be

reduced with proper treatment and preventive measures.

82. Can hemorrhoids change color?
External hemorrhoids may appear purple or blue if thrombosed due to blood accumulation.

83. Can hemorrhoids cause fatigue?
Hemorrhoids themselves do not cause fatigue, but chronic bleeding may lead to anemia, which may cause fatigue.

84. Can hemorrhoids cause vomiting?
Hemorrhoids themselves do not cause vomiting. However, if you experience vomiting along with hemorrhoid symptoms, it could indicate another medical condition that needs attention.

85. Can hemorrhoids cause burning?
Yes, hemorrhoids can cause burning, especially during bowel movements or cleansing, due to irritation of the skin and mucous membranes.

86. Can hemorrhoids cause acute pain?
Yes, hemorrhoids, especially if they are thrombosed or if there is a fissure, can cause acute and intense pain in the anal area.

87. Can hemorrhoids cause pain when walking?
Large or thrombosed hemorrhoids may cause pain when walking due to increased pressure in the anal area.

88. Can hemorrhoids cause pain when sitting?
Yes, external or prolapsed hemorrhoids can cause pain or discomfort when sitting, especially on hard surfaces.

89. Can hemorrhoids cause itching?
Yes, itching is a common symptom of hemorrhoids, especially if there is irritation or discharge in the anal area.

90. Can hemorrhoids cause itching in other areas of the body?
Hemorrhoids generally cause itching in the anal area, but not in other parts of the body. Itching in other regions may be due to a different cause.

91. Can hemorrhoids cause a feeling of urgency to evacuate?
Yes, hemorrhoids can cause a feeling of fullness or urgency to have a bowel movement due to swelling and pressure in the anal area.

92. Can hemorrhoids affect sex life?
Hemorrhoids can affect sex life, causing discomfort during intercourse or reducing sexual desire due to pain. Discussing any concerns with a physician is essential to finding appropriate solutions.

93. Can hemorrhoids cause pain during sexual intercourse?
Yes, especially if they are external or prolapsed, as they may cause pain or discomfort in the anal region during intercourse.

94. Can hemorrhoids cause fecal incontinence?
Hemorrhoids themselves do not usually cause fecal incontinence, but damage or weakness of the anal sphincter due to surgical procedures to remove them may contribute to it.

95. Can hemorrhoids cause abdominal pain?
Hemorrhoids usually do not cause abdominal pain. However, if abdominal symptoms occur, it is essential to consult a physician to rule out other conditions.

96. Can hemorrhoids cause abdominal cramps?
Hemorrhoids themselves do not cause abdominal cramps, but the associated constipation can cause abdominal discomfort.

97. Can hemorrhoids cause a foul odor?
Hemorrhoids do not cause odor; discharge or insufficient hygiene in the affected area can lead to an unpleasant odor. Maintaining good hygiene can help prevent this problem.

98. Can hemorrhoids cause inflammation in other parts of the body?
Hemorrhoids usually do not cause inflammation in other parts of the body, as they are a localized condition in the anal area.

99. Can hemorrhoids cause constipation?
Hemorrhoids do not cause constipation, but pain and discomfort during bowel movements may cause a person to avoid going to the bathroom, which could make constipation worse.

100. Can hemorrhoids cause gas or abdominal bloating?
Hemorrhoids do not directly cause gas or abdominal bloating, but associated constipation may contribute to these symptoms.

101. Can hemorrhoids cause pain in the coccyx?
Although hemorrhoids do not directly cause pain in the coccyx, general discomfort in the anal region may radiate and be

felt in the coccyx area.

102. Can hemorrhoids affect the quality of sleep?
Yes, the pain, itching, or discomfort caused by hemorrhoids can affect the quality of sleep in some people.

103. Can hemorrhoids cause anal itching?
Yes, anal itching is a common symptom of hemorrhoids due to irritation of the skin around the anus.

104. Can hemorrhoids cause nausea?
It is not common for hemorrhoids to cause nausea. A healthcare provider should evaluate Nausea as a symptom of another condition.

105. Can hemorrhoids cause weight loss?
Hemorrhoids do not usually cause weight loss. However, if unexplained weight loss occurs, it is essential to consult a physician.

106. Can hemorrhoids cause dizziness?
Hemorrhoids do not cause dizziness. If dizziness occurs, it may be a symptom of another condition and should be evaluated by a healthcare provider.

107. Can hemorrhoids cause leg pain?
Not directly, but leg pain could be related to circulatory problems that also affect hemorrhoids.

108. Can hemorrhoids cause back problems?
Although hemorrhoids do not cause back problems, their pain and discomfort may affect posture and indirectly contribute to back discomfort.

109. Can hemorrhoids cause urinary problems?
Hemorrhoids do not usually cause urinary problems, but discomfort or pain in the anal area may make urination difficult in some cases.

110. Can hemorrhoids cause fluid retention?
Hemorrhoids do not cause fluid retention. The retention may be related to other medical or dietary problems.

111. What is the Doppler treatment for hemorrhoids?
Doppler treatment uses ultrasound to identify and ligate the arteries that supply blood to the hemorrhoids, reducing their size.

112. When is surgery recommended for hemorrhoids?
Surgery may be recommended when hemorrhoids are large, very painful, or when less invasive treatments have not been effective.

113. What type of anesthesia is used in hemorrhoid surgery?
Hemorrhoid surgery can be performed under local, regional, or general anesthesia, depending on the procedure and the patient's and surgeon's preferences.

114. What are the surgical treatment options?
Surgical options include hemorrhoidectomy, stapled hemorrhoidopexy and transanal hemorrhoidal dearterialization, each with different indications and recovery times.

115. What is a hemorrhoidectomy?
A hemorrhoidectomy is a surgical procedure to remove hemorrhoids, generally recommended for severe or recurrent cases.

116. What type of anesthesia is used for a hemorrhoidectomy?
Depending on the case and the surgeon's recommendation, a hemorrhoidectomy may be performed under local, regional, or general anesthesia.

117. What postoperative care is necessary after a hemorrhoidectomy?
Care may include keeping the area clean and dry, taking analgesics as prescribed, avoiding straining, and following a fiber-rich diet to facilitate bowel movements.

118. What is mucosal folding for treating hemorrhoids?
Mucosal folding is a surgical procedure in which excess mucosal tissue is removed and prolapsed hemorrhoids are repositioned within the anus.

119. What is a stapled hemorrhoidopexy or Longo technique?
Stapled hemorrhoidopexy is a surgical procedure that uses a circular stapler to reposition and secure prolapsed hemorrhoids in their original place inside the rectum, reducing their size and symptoms.

120. What is transanal hemorrhoidal dearterialization?
THD is a procedure that consists of ligating the arteries that

supply blood to hemorrhoids, reducing their size and symptoms without removing the hemorrhoidal tissue.

121. What is the laser for the treatment of hemorrhoids?
Laser treatment uses laser energy to reduce or eliminate hemorrhoidal tissue, offering a less invasive alternative to traditional surgery.

122. What types of non-surgical procedures are available?
Nonsurgical procedures include rubber band ligation, sclerotherapy, infrared coagulation and cryotherapy, among others, which are designed to reduce the size of hemorrhoids.

123. What is rubber band ligation for hemorrhoids?
Rubber band ligation is a procedure in which a band is placed around the base of an internal hemorrhoid to cut off its blood supply, causing it to dry up and fall off.

124. What is sclerotherapy for hemorrhoids?
Sclerotherapy is a treatment in which a chemical solution is injected into hemorrhoids to shrink them by scarring the affected veins. It is an option for internal hemorrhoids that do not respond to conservative treatments.

125. What is infrared photocoagulation for hemorrhoids?
Infrared photocoagulation is a treatment that uses heat to coagulate proteins in the blood vessels of hemorrhoids, reducing their size.

126. What is cryotherapy for hemorrhoids?
Cryotherapy is a less common treatment that uses extreme cold to destroy hemorrhoidal tissue. However, it is not as widely used as other treatments because of its risks and potential complications.

127. What is bipolar coagulation for hemorrhoids?
Bipolar coagulation is a procedure that uses electrical current to coagulate the blood vessels of hemorrhoids, reducing their size and relieving symptoms.

128. Can hemorrhoids return after treatment?
Yes, hemorrhoids can return if underlying risk factors, such as chronic constipation or excessive straining, are not adequately managed after treatment.

SUGGESTED PRACTICAL PLAN

If you're dealing with hemorrhoids, here you'll find a practical and comprehensive guide to support you throughout your recovery process. This plan outlines key steps to relieve symptoms, prevent recurrence, and enhance your quality of life. It's time to take the first step toward your well-being!

▸ **Understand the Cause:** Identifying the possible reasons behind your hemorrhoids is a crucial first step. Pinpointing and addressing the triggering factors is essential to preventing the problem from returning. In the chapter "Hemorrhoids," review the sections "Causes" and "Symptoms Reduction and Prevention" to gain a clear and actionable understanding.

▸ **Support Your Recovery with Supplements:** The dietary supplements mentioned in the next chapter can greatly aid your healing process. Selecting the right supplement can make a meaningful difference in alleviating symptoms and accelerating recovery. Explore the available options and choose the one that's best suited to your needs. Your body will thank you!

▸ **Take Advantage of Herbal Remedies:** Many medicinal plants and herbal therapy recipes, highlighted in the chapter "Medicinal Plants", have been proven effective at reducing symptoms and speeding up recovery. Never underestimate the healing power of nature in your journey to better health.

▸ **Nutrition:** Your diet plays a vital role in managing hemorrhoids. Understanding which foods can help and which may aggravate your symptoms is critical. Refer to the chapters "Foods That Transform" and "Juices and Smoothies," where you'll find over 50 recipes tailored to support your recovery, alongside an assortment of juices specifically designed for this condition.

▸ **Identify and Eliminate Allergens:** Food allergens can exacerbate symptoms. Consider removing a specific food from your diet for at least 15 days to identify whether it is causing harm. Common culprits include gluten, dairy, and pork, but always pay attention to how your body responds.

▸ **Review Your Medication**: If you suspect that any medications you're taking (for any health condition) might be aggravating your hemorrhoids or causing new symptoms, consult your doctor. It's essential to evaluate whether an adjustment to your treatment could provide relief.

▸ **Lifestyle Adjustments**: Adopting healthy daily habits can play a crucial role in significantly reducing symptoms and preventing their recurrence. In the section "Symptoms Reduction and Prevention" of the chapter "Hemorrhoids," you'll discover practical and effective strategies to seamlessly integrate into your routine.

▸ **Stay Active**: Engaging in regular exercise enhances circulation, which often helps relieve pressure on the veins and supports the recovery process. Incorporate moderate physical activities—such as walking, swimming, or dancing—into your lifestyle to experience positive changes in the affected area.

Additional Resources
If you're managing other health concerns such as constipation, varicose veins, or SIBO, my other books may be of interest. They provide practical and natural strategies for addressing these conditions. Here are the titles that may offer further guidance:

▸ **CONSTIPATION**. Foods, Supplements & Herbs
▸ **SIBO**: Foods, Supplements & Herbs
▸ **VARICOSE VEINS**. Foods, Supplements & Herbs

This Is Your Time to Act!
This guide equips you with the tools to address hemorrhoids from multiple angles. By following these recommendations, you can effectively manage symptoms, prevent future flare-ups, and enhance your overall quality of life.

Start your journey to well-being today!

NUTRITIONAL SUPPLEMENTS

"Health is not everything, but without it, everything else is nothing"
(Arthur Schopenhauer)

Nutritional supplements have become a valuable ally in the pursuit of better health and an enhanced quality of life. These options—available in various user-friendly formats such as tablets, capsules, powders, or easily consumable liquids—are purposefully designed to complement your daily nutrition by delivering essential nutrients that can be challenging to obtain through regular meals alone. Packed with powerful components like vitamins, minerals, amino acids, antioxidants, and other bioactive compounds, these supplements are expertly formulated in precise proportions to meet the unique needs of every individual—even when the demands are high. Whether you're navigating restrictive diets, facing nutritional gaps, or coping with increased physical or mental demands, supplements can provide the extra support your body needs.

Beyond simply filling in nutritional gaps, supplements offer an array of tailored benefits to suit diverse lifestyles and health challenges. They can help boost energy, improve physical performance, support those managing fast-paced lives, and provide practical solutions for staying balanced and resilient. Their significance often becomes even more apparent during times of illness, specific health conditions, or chronic issues. In these situations, supplements do more than complement a diet—they can actively help restore altered functions, ease symptoms, and assist in more complex recovery processes. They serve as companions in the pursuit of health, helping you sustain and rebuild your vitality.

Effectively integrating supplements into your routine requires thoughtful use grounded in science and, when needed, professional guidance. By understanding their benefits and approaching them with care, supplements can evolve into powerful tools for improving your overall well-being in a sustainable and meaningful way. Remember—every step you take toward caring for your body is a step closer to feeling stronger, more energized, and more capable of facing life's challenges with confidence.

Take that step today. Your path to better health begins with small but impactful choices!

Essential Precautions

Understanding the risks associated with supplements is vital, as they can sometimes cause side effects, have contraindications, or interact with medications. It's important to thoroughly review the potential adverse effects detailed at the end of this chapter. Take a moment to assess your overall health and avoid any supplements that could conflict with the medications you're currently taking or exacerbate existing medical conditions. Prioritizing this step ensures a safer and more effective approach to improving your well-being.

Nutritional Supplements and Hemorrhoids

If you're dealing with the discomfort caused by hemorrhoids, I want you to know that there are effective ways to ease this situation. This chapter has been thoughtfully crafted for you, providing a clear and practical guide to help improve your daily life. We'll explore how nutritional supplements can serve as valuable allies, assisting you in not only reducing symptoms but also restoring your overall well-being.

In recent years, our understanding of how nutrition profoundly impacts health has grown significantly. From managing digestive disorders to improving emotional well-being, paying attention to what we consume remains one of the most effective ways to transform our health. Within this context, nutritional supplements have emerged as valuable and accessible tools to support the body, particularly when addressing uncomfortable conditions like hemorrhoids, which can greatly affect both physical comfort and emotional balance.

With this in mind, you'll find here a carefully curated list of supplements that could make a meaningful difference in your daily routine. Each recommendation is tailored to promote digestive health and alleviate the symptoms that trouble you the most. Additionally, the information is organized in a simple, alphabetical format, making it convenient to locate what you need quickly. Because when it comes to your well-being, even small actions can lead to significant improvements.

Aloe vera

Aloe vera, also known as Sabila, is a plant with medicinal properties. It has been traditionally used to treat various skin conditions and is also beneficial for relieving hemorrhoids.

Aloe vera gel contains active compounds with anti-inflammatory, analgesic, and healing properties. These properties help reduce inflammation, relieve pain, and promote the healing of hemorrhoids.

To use aloe in the treatment of hemorrhoids, you can follow these steps:

1. Make sure you get pure, high-quality aloe vera gel. You can find it in herbalists, health food stores, or pharmacies.

2. Clean the affected area with warm water and gently pat dry with a clean towel.

3. Apply a small amount of aloe vera gel directly to the hemorrhoids.

4. Gently massage the gel into the skin until completely absorbed.

Recommended dosage:
The recommended dose is usually 250 to 600 mg per day.

Posology:
For better absorption, it is recommended that you take it on an empty stomach, preferably in the morning or during the day.

Average action time:
The average time it takes to notice improvement can vary, but it usually occurs after weeks to months of continuous use.

Maximum recommended time of continuous use:
Continued use is generally considered safe for more than six months, but it is advisable to consult a specialist to determine the appropriate duration for your needs.

Blueberries

Blueberries have several health benefits and help treat

hemorrhoids.

Although there is no specific dosage for blueberry consumption for hemorrhoids, a general average dosage is suggested to obtain the benefits.

▸ Anti-inflammatory properties: They contain antioxidants and anti-inflammatory compounds that help reduce the inflammation and discomfort associated with hemorrhoids.

▸ Improved blood circulation: Regular consumption of blueberries helps to improve blood circulation, which is essential for alleviating hemorrhoids, often linked to circulation issues.

▸ High fiber: Blueberries are rich in fiber, which helps prevent constipation, a common risk factor for hemorrhoids. Fiber helps keep stools soft and facilitates regular bowel movements.

Posology:
To enjoy the benefits of blueberries for hemorrhoids, you can include them in your diet in the following ways:

▸ Consume fresh blueberries: You can eat them alone as a snack or add them to your smoothies, yogurts, or salads.

▸ Consume frozen blueberries: If fresh blueberries are not available, frozen blueberries are also a nutritious option. Thaw them and use them in your favorite recipes.

▸ Consume cranberry juice: Another way to reap the benefits of this fruit is to consume pure, unsweetened juice. Be sure to choose a high-quality juice without additives.

Flax Seeds

Flaxseeds, also known as linseeds, are an excellent source of fiber and omega-3 fatty acids. Here are some of the benefits they can provide for hemorrhoid management:

▸ High fiber content: They are an excellent source of dietary fiber, both soluble and insoluble. Fiber helps prevent constipation and promotes healthy digestion by keeping stools soft and facilitating their passage through the digestive system. This relieves straining during bowel movements and reduces pressure on rectal veins, which benefits people with hemorrhoids.

▸ Anti-inflammatory properties: They contain omega-3 fatty acids, which have anti-inflammatory properties. These properties help reduce inflammation and discomfort associated with hemorrhoids.

▸ Lubrication and constipation relief: Flax seeds contain mucilage that can absorb water and form a gel-like substance. This substance helps lubricate the intestines and promotes bowel regularity, which benefits people with hemorrhoids.

Recommended dosage:
The recommended dosage may vary depending on the source and individual needs. However, the recommended dosage is 1 to 2 tablespoons of flaxseeds daily. To obtain the benefits, it is suggested that flax seeds be ground before consumption, as this facilitates their digestion and absorption by the body.

Posology:
Flaxseeds can be added to the diet in several ways:

▸ Mix them in smoothies, yogurts, or cereals.
▸ Add them to baked goods such as bread or cookies.
▸ Use them in pancake or muffin recipes.

It is important to note that flaxseeds should be consumed with sufficient liquid to avoid intestinal obstruction.

Horse Chestnut

Horse chestnut (Aesculus hippocastanum) has traditionally been used as a natural remedy for hemorrhoids due to its anti-inflammatory and venotonic properties. Here are some benefits associated with its use:

▸ Reducing inflammation: It contains compounds such as aescin, which help reduce inflammation in hemorrhoids. This relieves symptoms such as pain, itching and swelling.

▸ Strengthening blood vessels: Horse chestnut extract strengthens blood vessels and improves their elasticity. This is beneficial for hemorrhoids, which are caused by dilation of the veins in the anal area.

▸ Improved blood circulation: It also improves blood circulation, which is essential for maintaining good venous health. Increased blood flow helps reduce clot formation and promotes faster recovery.

Recommended Dosage:
Generally, 300 to 600 mg of standardized extract (20% to 25% escin) is taken daily, which can be divided into smaller doses throughout the day.

Posology:
Taking two or three doses with meals throughout the day is usually recommended to improve gastrointestinal tolerance and absorption.

Average Action Initiation Time:
Its effects are generally observed within 1 to 2 weeks of continuous use.

Maximum Time of Continuous Use:
Continued use should be, at most, a period of 3 to 4 months. After this time, it is advisable to take a break or consult your physician and re-evaluate the need for continued treatment.

Omega-3

Its anti-inflammatory properties and cardiovascular health benefits are beneficial in managing hemorrhoids. Although there is no average recommended dosage specific to hemorrhoids, there are general guidelines for omega-3 consumption:

▸ Anti-inflammatory properties: Anti-inflammatory properties help reduce inflammation and discomfort related to hemorrhoids. Decreasing the inflammatory response relieves the symptoms associated with this condition.

▸ Improved blood circulation: This benefits cardiovascular health and promotes better circulation. It is especially beneficial for people with hemorrhoids, as these are often related to circulation problems.

▸ Promoting bowel health: This helps maintain bowel health and prevent constipation. Softer, more regular stools reduce pressure on rectal veins and decrease the risk of developing or worsening hemorrhoids.

Recommended dosage:
The recommended dosage ranges from 500 to 4000 mg daily, depending on the product's concentration of EPA (eicosa-

pentaenoic acid) and DHA (docosahexaenoic acid) and individual needs.

Posology:
It is recommended to be taken to facilitate absorption, preferably with a meal containing some fat. Depending on personal preference, it can be taken in the morning, afternoon, or evening.

Average action time:
The time of onset of action may vary, but the effect usually appears after a few weeks to a few months of continuous use.

Maximum recommended time of continuous use:
There is no established maximum time for continuous use. Suppose it is planned to be used for more than six months. In that case, it is recommended that you follow the manufacturer's instructions or consult a specialist, especially for people with coagulation disorders.

Psyllium

Psyllium, or Plantago ovata, is widely recognized for its digestive health benefits, including hemorrhoid relief. Here are some benefits associated with its use:

▸ Relief from constipation: Psyllium fiber is a soluble fiber that absorbs water in the intestine. This helps soften the stool and facilitate its passage through the digestive system. This is especially beneficial for people who suffer from constipation, as straining during bowel movements can worsen hemorrhoids.

▸ Improved stool consistency: Psyllium fiber in the diet promotes the formation of softer, bulkier stools. This helps prevent straining during bowel movements and reduces hemorrhoid irritation.

▸ Regulation of intestinal transit: It acts as a natural regulator of intestinal transit. It helps prevent constipation and diarrhea, properly balancing intestinal function.

Recommended dosage:
As for the average recommended dosage for psyllium fiber in treating hemorrhoids, following the manufacturer's directions is essential. However, here are some general guidelines:

‣ Psyllium powder: The recommended dose is approximately 5 grams (one teaspoon) mixed with water or juice once or twice daily. It is essential to drink enough water after taking it to avoid dehydration.

‣ Psyllium capsules: The recommended dosage generally ranges from 2 to 6 capsules per day, depending on the concentration and instructions of the specific product.

Vitamin E

It is an essential nutrient with antioxidant properties, providing overall health and wellness benefits. Here are some of the benefits for hemorrhoids:

‣ Antioxidant properties: Vitamin E is known for its antioxidant activity, which helps protect cells from free radical damage. This benefits hemorrhoids, as it helps reduce inflammation and promotes tissue health.

‣ Promotes wound healing: Vitamin E promotes healing and tissue regeneration. Although hemorrhoids are not open wounds, they may be associated with minor injuries or irritations in the anal area. Vitamin E helps accelerate healing and reduce discomfort.

‣ Immune system support: Vitamin E plays a vital role in the functioning of the immune system. Maintaining a healthy immune system is essential for managing hemorrhoids, as it helps prevent infections and promotes the body's proper response to stress.

Average Recommended Dose:
It ranges from 100 to 400 IU (international units) per day. Higher doses may be used under medical supervision in some cases.

Posology:
Since it is a fat-soluble vitamin, it should be taken in one or two doses with meals containing fat to improve its absorption.

Action Initiation Time:
Generally, antioxidant effects usually begin to be noticed within 1 to 3 weeks of continuous use, although specific benefits may take longer to become evident.

Maximum Time of Continuous Use:
Vitamin E is generally safe for long-term use. However, 400 IU per day should be continuously exceeded without medical supervision. Some experts suggest continued use for up to 1 year, but it is essential to consult a healthcare professional to determine the appropriate duration based on your needs.

Witch Hazel

Witch hazel (Hamamelis virginiana) is a plant that has long been used to treat hemorrhoids due to its astringent and anti-inflammatory properties. Here are some benefits associated with its use:

‣ Reduction of inflammation: Witch hazel contains compounds known as tannins, which have anti-inflammatory properties. These tannins help reduce inflammation and relieve hemorrhoid symptoms, such as pain and swelling.

‣ Relief from discomfort: It relieves pain associated with hemorrhoids, such as itching and burning. Its astringent properties help soothe and protect irritated skin.

‣ Improved blood circulation: Witch hazel also helps to improve blood circulation in the affected area. This benefits hemorrhoids, as poor circulation can contribute to their formation and worsen symptoms.

Recommended dosage:
As for the average recommended dosage in the treatment of hemorrhoids, the following guidelines can be followed:

‣ Witch hazel tincture: It is recommended that a small amount of witch hazel tincture be applied directly to the hemorrhoids with a cotton ball or clean cloth several times a day as needed.

‣ Witch hazel ointment: Witch hazel ointments are available in cream or ointment form. Follow the manufacturer's instructions for how often and how much to apply.

Adverse Effects, Contraindications, and Interactions

Before adding the recommended supplements to your routine, it is crucial to understand the potential side effects, contra-indications, and interactions that may affect your health. Take the time to thoroughly review this section to ensure their safe and responsible use.

Aloe Vera

▸ **Side effects**: When consumed orally, aloe may cause diarrhea, abdominal cramping, and electrolyte imbalances. Topical use may cause skin irritation, redness, or allergies in some people.

▸ **Contraindications**: Aloe vera is contraindicated in people with intestinal obstruction, appendicitis, inflammatory bowel disease, severe kidney and heart disease, as well as during pregnancy and lactation.

▸ **Interactions**: It may interact with antidiabetic medications, diuretics and drugs that affect the cardiovascular system. Please consult your doctor or pharmacist before combining it with any medication.

Blueberries

▸ **Side Effects**: Cranberry consumption is generally considered safe, and no significant side effects have been reported. However, it may cause stomach upset or diarrhea in some sensitive people.

▸ **Contraindications**: No specific contraindications have been identified.

▸ **Interactions**: No significant drug interactions have been reported. However, it is always advisable to consult your doctor before combining it with any medication.

Flax seed

▸ **Side effects**: Flaxseed consumption in moderate amounts is generally considered safe. However, if not enough liquid is consumed, it may cause gas, stomach upset, and even intestinal obstruction in some people.

▸ **Contraindications**: People with intestinal obstruction, severe gastrointestinal disorders, or known allergy to flaxseeds should avoid consumption.

▸ **Interactions**: No significant drug interactions have been reported. However, it is always advisable to consult a health professional before combining it with any medication.

Horse Chestnut

‣ **Side effects**: It may cause gastrointestinal discomfort, such as nausea and stomach upset. Rarely, it may produce effects such as vomiting, diarrhea and dizziness.

‣ **Contraindications**: It is not recommended in people with liver or kidney disease, coagulation disorders, pregnancy, lactation, or allergy to this plant.

‣ **Interactions**: Horse chestnut may interact with anticoagulants and antiplatelet medications. Please consult your doctor before using it in combination with these drugs.

Omega-3

‣ **Side effects**: The most common side effects are fishy taste, fishy belching and stomach upset. In high doses, it may also increase the risk of bleeding.

‣ **Contraindications**: Caution is advised in people with bleeding disorders, diabetes, coagulation disorders, or allergies to fish or shellfish. Pregnant or lactating women should also consult a physician before taking omega-3 supplements.

‣ **Interactions**: It may interact with anticoagulants, antiplatelets and blood pressure medications. Please consult your doctor before combining it with any medication.

Psyllium

‣ **Side effects**: Psyllium fiber may cause some people to experience bloating, gas, and abdominal discomfort. Drinking enough water is also essential to avoid intestinal obstruction.

‣ **Contraindications**: Not recommended in people with intestinal obstruction, difficulty swallowing, or esophageal problems.

‣ **Interactions**: Psyllium fiber may decrease the absorption of some medications, such as tricyclic antidepressants, anticonvulsants and diabetes medications. Therefore, it is recommended that medications and Psyllium fiber be taken at an adequate time interval.

Vitamin E

‣ **Side effects**: Vitamin E is generally well tolerated in average doses. However, high doses may increase the risk of bleeding and hemorrhage and cause stomach upset in some people.

‣ **Contraindications**: Caution is advised in people with bleeding disorders, diabetes, coagulation disorders, or allergy to vitamin E.

‣ **Interactions**: It may interact with anticoagulants and antiplatelet medications. Please consult your doctor before combining it with any medication.

Witch Hazel

‣ **Side effects**: Topical use of witch hazel may cause skin irritation or allergies in some people.

‣ **Contraindications**: Its use should be avoided in people with known allergies to this plant.

‣ **Interactions**: No significant drug interactions have been reported. However, it is always advisable to consult a physician before combining it with any medication.

FOODS THAT TRANSFORM

"When food is bad, medicine does not work. When food is good, medicine is not necessary" (Ayurvedic proverb)

Throughout history, our diet has undergone profoundly radical changes, sharply diverging from the habits of our ancestors. Millions of years ago, early humans shaped their diet around what they could gather or hunt, relying on fresh and raw foods provided by their environment. The emergence of agriculture and livestock farming marked the beginning of a new era of human nutrition, further accelerated by the Industrial Revolution. However, it is important to recognize that while our dietary habits have evolved drastically, our genetics have remained virtually unchanged.

Over time, foods such as dairy products, grains, refined sugars, and vegetable oils were introduced, alongside the rise of intensive meat production. These innovations have made meals more accessible and convenient, yet they have also led to significant changes in nutritional composition. Furthermore, advances in food preservation and culinary techniques gave rise to new methods of storage and preparation, which inevitably impacted food quality.

In recent years, an alarming trend has surfaced: modern diets have become dominated by ultra-processed foods, contributing to the widespread increase in chronic illnesses. Conditions such as obesity, type 2 diabetes, hypertension, and a variety of cardiovascular and digestive disorders have all been closely linked to this dietary shift. Why is this happening? Primarily because ultra-processed foods are heavily laden with refined carbohydrates, unhealthy fats, added sugars, chemical additives, and low-quality vegetable oils. Even meats and other animal products from intensive farming systems are often filled with substances harmful to health. These processed foods have largely replaced traditional diets, which were built on fresh and natural ingredients, disrupting the equilibrium that once fostered optimal well-being among our ancestors.

Nonetheless, there is hope for reversing this trend: small yet thoughtful changes to our eating habits can have a significant impact on our health. Returning to a balanced, nutrient-rich way of eating, centered on fresh, whole foods, is essential for establishing a strong foundation for wellness. Integrating fruits, vegetables, root vegetables, legumes, nuts, and seeds into the diet is a powerful step toward revitalizing the way we nourish ourselves. Despite this, one major challenge persists: the consumption of these natural, unprocessed foods remains astonishingly low in many parts of the world.

Choosing a lifestyle rooted in mindful eating not only helps prevent diseases associated with poor dietary habits but also rejuvenates the body and mind. By prioritizing real, wholesome foods and cutting back on ultra-processed options, we can cultivate a healthier, more balanced, and fulfilling life. Now is the time to rediscover the transformative power of a healthy diet–not as a form of restriction, but as an act of self-care. Your health deserves that commitment!

Understanding the Link Between Nutrition and Health

How often have you asked yourself if what you eat truly supports your well-being? The relationship between nutrition and health is far deeper than we commonly realize. Understanding which foods promote wellness and which ones to avoid, tailored to your specific needs, is a powerful step toward improving your quality of life. This isn't a new concept; it has been examined and revered for centuries. Since ancient times, cultures around the world have recognized the therapeutic value of nutrition as a means to heal, strengthen, and sustain the body, leaving us a profound legacy of wisdom.

Traditional medical systems–such as Traditional Chinese Medicine, the practices of ancient Egypt, Greece, and Rome, Ayurveda in India, and indigenous healing methods across the Americas–delved into the restorative potential of natural foods. These practices emphasized the idea that food does much more than nourish; it can protect, alleviate discomfort, and even heal the body.

For many years, these age-old principles were often dismissed by conventional medicine as unscientific. Yet, modern research has gradually confirmed what our ancestors intuitively under-stood: the foods we eat directly affect not only our physical health but also our emotional well-being. Today, scientific studies continue to uncover compounds in food with therapeutic properties that help prevent diseases, reduce symptoms, and promote overall health.

Researchers have spent decades analyzing how certain foods strengthen the body and protect against chronic illnesses, identifying dietary patterns in populations with low disease rates that differ significantly from those in less healthy communities. These studies reveal the decisive role specific nutrients play in promoting vitality and longevity, with certain foods offering unique benefits such as anti-inflammatory properties to manage joint pain and chronic discomfort, antimicrobial effects to bolster immune defenses, anticoagulant actions to support cardio-vascular health, antihypertensive abilities to regulate blood pressure, and mood-enhancing compounds that alleviate anxiety while fostering emotional resilience.

What you choose to eat influences not only your daily energy but also your capacity to recover, fend off illness, and pursue a fulfilling life. On the flip side, a poor diet or reliance on unhealthy foods can exacerbate health problems, intensify symptoms, and undermine overall well-being.

The encouraging part? Every day offers the chance to make dietary choices that lead to better health. While external factors like pollution or environmental changes may remain out of your control, your diet is a fundamental tool for self-care. Each ingredient on your plate carries the potential to positively impact both your physical and mental health.

Learning which foods are best for your unique needs–and understanding which ones may harm your health–can empower you to find balance and achieve a healthier, more vibrant lifestyle. Nutrition, humanity's earliest form of medicine, is not just a pathway to wellness but also a connection to our roots, equipping us for a future filled with possibilities.

I invite you to explore how nutrition can become your strongest ally in easing ailments, building resilience, and fostering happiness. Are you ready to embrace this journey of discovery and transformation? Your well-being is within your control, and every meal is a chance to create a life of greater health and vitality. Start today: Nourish your body, refresh your mind, and live fully.

Foods and Hemorrhoids

If you are experiencing an acute hemorrhoidal crisis, it is essential to pay close attention to your diet, as it can have a significant impact on your recovery. During such episodes, it is crucial to follow the recommendations provided in the subchapter "**Foods and Beverages to Avoid During Hemorrhoidal Crises**" and strictly limit the consumption of foods that are not advised. However, outside of the most severe episodes, occasional consumption of these items in small quantities is unlikely to cause significant harm if practiced in moderation.

A key factor in managing this condition is maintaining adequate hydration. Drinking enough water throughout the day is essential not only for overall health but also for softening stools. This helps reduce straining during bowel movements, a vital step to prevent further irritation or worsening of hemorrhoids.

If you experience constipation or excessively hard stools, which can exacerbate the condition, you may consider temporarily using stimulant laxatives or stool softeners for a duration of 1 to 7 days. These measures can provide relief from constipation while your body adjusts to a gradual increase in fiber and fluid intake.

Attending to your diet and staying well-hydrated, particularly during times of heightened sensitivity, can make a significant difference in how effectively you manage this condition and in your overall comfort. Your body will thank you!

Foods and Beverages to Avoid During Hemorrhoidal Crises

Diet plays a pivotal role in managing hemorrhoids, particularly during a crisis. Certain foods and beverages can exacerbate symptoms by increasing irritation, inflammation, or the strain required during bowel movements. Therefore, it is crucial to identify and avoid anything that could aggravate the condition, facilitating a faster and more comfortable recovery.

Below is a detailed list of the primary foods and beverages that should ideally be avoided during episodes of acute hemorrhoidal crises. Adhering to these recommendations can significantly improve your well-being during periods of intense pain and discomfort.

‣ **Spicy foods**: Foods such as chili, bell pepper and curry can irritate hemorrhoids and increase the burning sensation and discomfort. It is advisable to avoid these foods or reduce their consumption.

‣ **Fatty foods**: Foods high in saturated or trans fats can worsen constipation and make it harder to pass stool, increasing pressure on hemorrhoidal veins. Avoiding fried foods, high-fat processed foods, fatty meats, and full-fat dairy products may help reduce symptoms.

‣ **Alcoholic beverages:** Drinking alcohol can dehydrate the body and make it difficult to pass stool, which can aggravate constipation and increase discomfort during a hemorrhoidal crisis. It is recommended to avoid or limit alcoholic beverages until symptoms have improved.

‣ **Coffee and caffeinated beverages:** Coffee and other caffeinated beverages, such as black tea and energy drinks, can act as diuretics and dehydrate the body. This can worsen constipation and increase pressure on hemorrhoidal veins. Reduce or eliminate your intake.

‣ **Processed and refined foods:** Processed foods, such as baked goods, canned foods and commercial snack foods, often contain high levels of salt, saturated fats and additives that can increase inflammation and discomfort in hemorrhoids. Fresh, natural foods like fruits, vegetables and whole grains are the best choices.

‣ **Carbonated beverages:** Carbonated drinks can cause bloating and gas, increasing pressure in the hemorrhoid area and causing additional discomfort. Avoiding or limiting the consumption of these beverages during a hemorrhoidal crisis is advisable.

‣ **Foods high in refined sugar:** Foods high in refined sugar, such as candy, cakes, cookies and sugary soft drinks, can contribute to constipation and worsen hemorrhoid symptoms. These foods are often low in fiber and can cause fluctuations in blood sugar levels, affecting bowel health.

‣ **Whole dairy products:** Whole dairy products, such as milk, cheese and butter, can contain high levels of saturated fats, which can hinder digestion and worsen constipation. The best option, especially during a hemorrhoidal crisis, is to opt for low-fat dairy or plant-based alternatives, such as almond or soy milk with no added sugar.

‣ **Red meat:** Red meat, especially when consumed in large amounts, can be challenging to digest and worsen constipation. It is also high in saturated fat, which can increase inflammation and pressure in hemorrhoidal veins. Reducing red meat consumption and opting for lean protein sources like chicken, fish, and legumes may help relieve symptoms.

‣ **Processed foods with additives**: Foods with additives, such as preservatives, artificial colorings and flavorings, can irritate the digestive system and increase inflammation in the hemorrhoid area. Reading food labels and avoiding foods with a long list of chemical ingredients is advisable.

‣ **Foods high in sodium**: Foods high in sodium, such as canned, fast, and processed foods, can contribute to fluid retention and constipation. Fluid retention can increase pressure in hemorrhoidal veins and worsen symptoms. It is recommended to limit sodium consumption and opt for low-salt options.

Healing Foods According to TCM

The ancient wisdom of Traditional Chinese Medicine (TCM) provides valuable insights into managing hemorrhoids through diet. According to this approach, certain foods are renowned for their powerful anti-inflammatory properties, which help reduce venous dilation–the primary cause of the pain and discomfort associated with this condition.

Moreover, these foods are especially rich in essential nutrients, including fiber, bioflavonoids, and vitamins A, B, C, and E, as well as minerals like zinc. These nutrients play a crucial role in strengthening venous walls, enhancing circulation, and minimizing the recurrence of hemorrhoids.

Below is a comprehensive, alphabetically organized list of foods recommended by TCM to optimize their healing benefits. Incorporating these foods into your daily diet can be a meaningful step toward recovery and restoring balance to your overall well-being.

Adzuki or Azuki bean (Phaseolus angularis)

For hemorrhoids and bleeding hemorrhoids:
Ingredients: 60 g of Adzuki beans and pork casing.

Preparation: Boil everything over low heat until it is well-cooked. Then, consume the broth for 4 to 6 days.

Precautions: According to TCM, excessive consumption may cause loss of body fluids and thinness due to its diuretic effect.

People who urinate frequently and in large quantities should consume it with caution.

Apricot (Prunus armeniaca)

Ingredients: 50 g apricot kernels, 50 g non-glutinous round rice.

Preparation: Grind the almonds and soak them in water for 2 hours. Extract the juice and boil it in 1.5 liters of water until only half a liter remains. Add the rice and prepare a soup. Consume this soup twice a day.

Precautions: According to Traditional Chinese Medicine (TCM), due to its hot nature, excessive consumption of apricots can cause hot ulcers, which can lead to blindness and alopecia. Therefore, the recommended amount should be consumed strictly. People who tend to have internal heat should avoid its consumption. The apricot kernel contains amygdalin, which, when ingested, is converted into hydrocyanic acid by enzymatic hydrolysis, a highly toxic substance that should also not be consumed in excess.

Cilantro or Coriander (Coriandrum sativum)

For hemorrhoids and rectal prolapse:
Ingredients: 500 grams of cilantro.

Preparation: Boil coriander in covered water. Once it boils, make an incision and wash the anal area.

You can crush the seeds and apply the paste to the affected area.

Fig (Ficus carica)

For hemorrhoids with pain and/or bleeding:
Ingredients: 2 fresh, unripe figs.

Preparation: Consume in the morning and evening.
You can also use the white juice to pluck the fig tree leaves and apply them to the area.

For hemorrhoids, rectal prolapse, and/or constipation:
Ingredients: 10 fresh or dried figs, a piece of pork casing. If they

are fresh, the figs are eaten first, and then the pork casing is cooked to drink the broth. If they are dried, they are eaten after cooking with the pork casing.

For hemorrhoids with pain:
Ingredients: several fig leaves.

Preparation: Boil the leaves and take a sitz bath with the liquid on the affected area.

Precautions: According to TCM, fresh fig is an excellent laxative, so it should not be consumed by people with very soft or liquid stools.

Kiwi Fruit (Actinidia chinensis)

Ingredients: 200 grams of fresh kiwi.

Preparation: Consume peeled and ground kiwis twice a day, in the morning and at night.

Precautions: According to TCM, Kiwis' cold nature may cause diarrhea if consumed excessively. They are especially contraindicated for people predisposed to diarrhea or with delicate stomachs.

Pumpkin (Cucurbita moschata)

For internal hemorrhoids:
Ingredients: 1 kilo of pumpkin seeds.

Preparation: Boil the seeds in water. After boiling, remove them from the fire without covering and proceed to make an incense and wash the anus. Perform this procedure twice a day for 5 days.

Precautions: According to TCM, pumpkins are warm and sweet so that excessive consumption may cause indigestion. People suffering from dysentery or jaundice should also consume them with caution.

Sesame (Sesamum indicum)

Ingredients: 100 grams of sesame seeds, 500 ml of water.

Preparation: Boil the sesame seeds and use the broth to wash the affected area.

Tofu

Ingredients: Half a slice of tofu, 1 teaspoon of sugar, and water.

Preparation: Place the tofu and sugar in a pot and add water to cover the tofu. Bring to a boil and then reduce the heat, and maintain this temperature for 5 minutes. Turn off the heat and remove the pot. Consume this preparation in the morning on an empty stomach.

Other Recommended Foods

In addition to the previously mentioned foods, there are others that can be particularly beneficial for managing hemorrhoids. Here are the details:

‣ **Apple Cider Vinegar**: Mix 2 teaspoons of apple cider vinegar with a glass of water and drink it 2 to 3 times a day. This simple remedy helps to improve blood circulation, relieve pressure on the veins, and reduce the risk of excessive bleeding associated with hemorrhoids.

‣ **Foods That Promote Healing**: Incorporate foods with healing and anti-inflammatory properties into your diet, including: Onions, ginger, garlic, and pineapple.

These foods contribute to tissue regeneration and enhance the recovery process.

‣ **Beneficial Vegetables**: Other highly beneficial foods include: Watercress, turnips, and parsley.

These vegetables, in addition to being light and nutritious, are rich in vitamins and minerals that strengthen vascular health and overall well-being. By including these foods in your daily routine, you'll support symptom relief and promote an improved quality of life while managing this condition.

Additional Topical Remedies

Here is a selection of natural topical treatments designed to ease both internal and external hemorrhoids. These remedies are simple to use and can effectively help reduce inflammation, pain, and itching associated with the condition.

For internal hemorrhoids:
Garlic
Apply this remedy at night before going to sleep. Peel a clove of garlic, completely removing its peel, and cut it into a suppository shape. Please insert it into the rectum, lubricating it with olive oil to facilitate insertion. Leave it overnight. The garlic clove will be expelled naturally during bowel movements. Garlic is very effective in reducing itching and inflammation.

Potato
Peel the potato, wash your hands well, and cut a small piece in the shape of a suppository. Insert it raw into the rectum. Apply this remedy 1 or 2 times a day.

For external hemorrhoids:
Castor Oil
If you have inflamed hemorrhoids, apply 4 or 5 drops of oil on the previously washed area. You can use it 3 times a day.

Garlic
Chop 3 or 4 garlic cloves and boil them in a cup of water for 10 minutes. Strain the garlic pieces and let the water cool. Take a gauze and soak it in the water. Apply it to the hemorrhoids. You can cool the water in the refrigerator for additional relief. Another way to apply it is to crush garlic, place the resulting paste on a gauze, and keep it in contact with the bumps for at least 5 minutes. After that time, remove the gauze and wash the area with plenty of warm or cold water.

Garlic, Bay Leaf and Cloves
Take 3 cloves of garlic, 2 bay leaves and 5 cloves. Boil half a liter of water. Add the crushed garlic, bay leaves and cloves when it boils. Let it simmer for about 15 to 20 minutes. Then, please remove it from the heat and let it cool down. Strain the mixture and reserve the liquid obtained. This liquid will serve as an ointment for various applications. To use it, pour a little gauze and apply it directly on the hemorrhoids, leaving it to act for 5 to 10 minutes.

Potato

Grate some potatoes and place them in the area for several minutes.

Tomato

Take a ripe tomato and cut it in half. Place it on the hemorrhoids and sit on it for 15 minutes, 1 or 2 times a day.

Recommended Foods and Beverages for Hemorrhoids

Maintaining a balanced diet rich in fiber is crucial for relieving hemorrhoid symptoms and enhancing overall digestive health. An appropriate diet can help prevent constipation, reduce inflammation, and promote smoother, more regular bowel movements. Below is a carefully curated selection of foods and beverages particularly beneficial for individuals suffering from hemorrhoids:

▸ **Sources of fiber**: Eating fiber-rich foods is essential for maintaining a healthy digestive tract and reducing strain during bowel movements. Options include fresh fruits such as apples, pears, bananas, and berries, and vegetables such as broccoli, spinach, carrots and squash. Whole grains such as brown rice, oatmeal, and whole wheat bread are also beneficial.

▸ **Legumes and beans**: Legumes, such as chickpeas, lentils and kidney beans, are excellent sources of fiber and protein. Adding them to salads, soups, or stews can help increase fiber intake and improve bowel regularity.

▸ **Water**: Staying hydrated is essential for hemorrhoid treatment. Drinking enough water helps soften the stool, reducing strain during bowel movements. It is recommended that you drink at least 8 glasses of water daily.

▸ **Nuts and seeds**: Nuts, such as walnuts and almonds, as well as chia and flax seeds, are rich in fiber and healthy fats. They can help promote healthy digestion and prevent constipation.

▸ **Yogurt and probiotic foods**: Probiotic foods like yogurt and kefir contain beneficial bacteria that can improve intestinal health. By maintaining a healthy balance of bacteria in the digestive tract, these foods may help relieve hemorrhoid symptoms.

‣ **Olive oil**: Extra virgin olive oil is a healthy choice for cooking and seasoning foods. It contains anti-inflammatory properties and can help soften stools.

How food is prepared is just as crucial as selecting the right ingredients. Ideally, you should choose simple cooking methods, such as steaming, grilling, or baking en papillote, as these retain nutrients more effectively and are generally healthier. While some foods may seem less advisable, it's not essential to eliminate them entirely; instead, focus on preparing them in a lighter, healthier manner by reducing fat and avoiding irritating condiments, making them more suitable and easier to digest.

Foods and Beverages to Limit or Avoid

Nutrition plays a fundamental role in managing hemorrhoids, as certain foods and beverages can exacerbate symptoms and impede recovery. Identifying items that may cause irritation or lead to constipation is crucial, and their consumption should be reduced or avoided altogether whenever possible. Below is a list of the key foods and beverages to limit or eliminate in order to support relief and promote healing:

‣ **Spicy food**: Spicy foods, such as chili peppers, hot tomato sauce and strong condiments, can irritate hemorrhoids and increase inflammation. It is advisable to avoid them or reduce their consumption to alleviate symptoms.

‣ **Processed foods**: Processed foods, such as sausages, fast foods and packaged snacks, are often rich in saturated fats and chemical additives. These foods can worsen constipation, which is a common trigger for hemorrhoids. Instead, it is recommended to opt for fresh, natural foods.

‣ **Alcoholic beverages**: Excessive alcohol consumption can dehydrate the body and make it difficult for the digestive system to function correctly. This can lead to increased constipation and aggravate hemorrhoids. It is crucial to reduce or avoid alcohol consumption and opt for healthier alternatives, such as water, herbal teas, or natural juices.

‣ **Caffeine**: Coffee and other caffeinated beverages, such as black tea and energy drinks, can act as diuretics and worsen dehydration and constipation. Limiting their consumption may be beneficial in managing hemorrhoids.

‣ **Foods high in saturated fats**: Saturated fats, found in foods such as red meat, full-fat dairy products and fried foods, can hinder digestion and increase pressure on hemorrhoidal veins. Opting for lean protein sources and healthy fats, such as fish, skinless poultry, nuts and avocados, may be a more favorable alternative.

‣ **Dairy**: Some people may experience lactose intolerance or sensitivity to dairy products, which can sometimes worsen hemorrhoid symptoms. If you notice that dairy worsens your symptoms, you may want to consider alternatives such as lactose-free milk, plant-based milk, or fermented dairy products, such as probiotic yogurt.

‣ **Foods high in sugar**: Foods and beverages high in refined sugars, such as sweets, cakes, soft drinks and commercial juices, can contribute to constipation and weight gain. Excess weight can put additional pressure on hemorrhoidal veins, worsening symptoms. It is advisable to limit the consumption of these foods and opt for healthier, low-sugar alternatives, such as fresh fruits.

‣ **Low-fiber foods**: Lack of fiber in the diet is a risk factor for constipation, which can aggravate hemorrhoids. It is crucial to avoid or reduce consumption of refined and processed foods, such as white bread, white rice and regular pasta, which are low in fiber. Instead, choose whole-grain foods like bread, brown rice, whole-wheat pasta, and fresh fruits and vegetables.

‣ **Irritating foods**: Some foods can irritate the lining of the digestive tract and worsen hemorrhoid symptoms. These foods include citrus fruits, such as oranges and lemons, tomatoes, and acidic foods. If you feel these foods are causing discomfort, reducing their consumption or avoiding them temporarily is advisable.

‣ **Foods that cause gas**: Some foods can cause intestinal gas and increase pressure in the anal area, which can aggravate hemorrhoid symptoms. These foods include legumes, such as beans, lentils, and chickpeas, and cruciferous vegetables, such as broccoli and cauliflower. If you experience discomfort from gas, you can reduce your consumption or look for alternative cooking methods that make them more digestible.

Adopting a healthy lifestyle is equally important. Complement your diet with regular physical activity, as it promotes better circulation and supports intestinal health. Avoid prolonged periods of sitting or standing, and prioritize gentle, meticulous hygiene in the anal area to prevent irritation. By integrating these habits into your routine, you'll not only help alleviate symptoms but also minimize the risk of recurrence or worsening in the future.

Cooking Techniques

Healthy cooking is essential for everyone, especially after the age of 40. Below are various cooking techniques along with their related health benefits and potential risks.

Healthier Ways of Cooking

‣ **Steaming**: Steaming is an excellent method for preserving nutrients, as it does not require the use of additional fats. It helps keep food tender and juicy while being a gentle cooking technique that does not contribute to the formation of harmful compounds.

‣ **Oven roasting**: Oven roasting is a healthy option that does not require added oils. Foods like vegetables, fish, and chicken can be roasted in the oven to create nutritious and flavorful meals.

‣ **Light sautéing**: This method involves quickly cooking food over high heat with a small amount of healthy oil, such as olive or coconut oil. Light sautéing helps maintain the food's texture and nutrients while cooking it efficiently.

‣ **Boiling**: Boiling is a healthy cooking method, particularly for vegetables. It preserves nutrients and creates a tender texture. However, it is crucial to avoid overcooking to minimize nutrient loss.

‣ **Baking**: Baking is an excellent way to prepare food without the need for added oils. Foods like fish, poultry, vegetables, and whole grains can be baked for healthy and flavorful dishes.

Less Healthy Ways of Cooking

‣ **Frying**: Frying involves submerging food in hot oil, which significantly increases its saturated fat and calorie content. Additionally, frying at high temperatures can produce harmful compounds that pose health risks.

‣ **Breading and battering**: Coating food in breading or batter increases its calorie and fat content. These coatings can absorb more oil during cooking, resulting in a less nutritious meal.

‣ **Creamy sauces and dressings:** Cream-based sauces and dressings often contain high levels of saturated fat and excess calories. These can contribute to inflammation and exacerbate pain.

‣ **Grilling at high temperatures:** Cooking food on the grill at high heat can generate harmful compounds, such as polycyclic aromatic hydrocarbons (PAHs) and heterocyclic amines (HCAs), which have been associated with an increased cancer risk. Additionally, grilled meats can produce inflammatory substances.

Remember, the way you cook food significantly impacts its nutritional value and its overall effects on your health. Choosing healthy cooking methods ensures you maximize the benefits of your meals while reducing potential negative effects.

Hemorrhoids Support: Easy and Tasty Recipes

Here is a thoughtfully curated collection of quick, simple, and delicious recipes designed to promote intestinal health and ease the symptoms of hemorrhoids. These recipes are not only nutritious but also help prevent future discomfort while encouraging healthy eating habits. Take care of yourself and enjoy the process!

Breakfast Options

1. Oatmeal with fruit: Prepare a bowl of oatmeal with low-fat milk and add fruit pieces such as bananas, berries, or apples. Avoid adding sugar and choose to sweeten with honey or stevia.

2. Green smoothie: Blend fresh spinach, pineapple chunks, cucumber, lemon juice and water in a blender. Add ice for a cooler, more refreshing consistency.

3. Avocado and egg toast: Toast a slice of whole wheat bread and add a layer of sliced avocado. Cook a scrambled or poached egg and place it on the avocado. Sprinkle with salt and pepper to taste.

4. Yogurt with seeds and fruits: For extra fiber, opt for plain unsweetened yogurt and add chia, flaxseed, or sunflower seeds. You can also add fruit pieces such as bananas, apples, or peaches.

5. Egg white omelet with vegetables: Prepare an omelet with egg whites and add vegetables such as spinach, mushrooms, tomatoes and onion. Cook over medium heat until ready.

6. Berry and spinach smoothie: Blend frozen berries (such as strawberries, blueberries, or raspberries) with fresh spinach, low-fat milk, and a tablespoon of nut or seed butter.

7. Oatmeal-banana pancakes: Blend flaked oatmeal, ripe banana, eggs, and cinnamon until smooth. Cook pancakes in a non-stick pan and serve with fresh fruit and a spoonful of honey.

8. Protein and fruit smoothie: Blend protein powder (ensure it's appropriate for your medical situation), low-fat milk, spinach, banana, and berries in a blender. Add ice for a cooler consistency.

9. Avocado and tomato toast: Toast a slice of whole wheat bread and add sliced avocado, sliced tomato and a little sea salt—season with black pepper and parsley.

Lunch Creations

1. Spinach and Salmon Salad: Combine fresh spinach with grilled salmon chunks, cherry tomatoes, cucumber and walnuts. Dress with olive oil, lemon juice, and a pinch of salt.

2. Chicken and Vegetable Wraps: Wrap grilled chicken breasts in a whole wheat tortilla. Add bell pepper strips, shredded carrots and lettuce leaves. Serve with a low-fat dip, such as herbed Greek yogurt.

3. Vegetable Soup: Prepare a comforting soup with low-sodium vegetable broth, adding carrots, zucchini, and peppers. For added flavor, add herbs such as parsley and thyme.

4. Quinoa and vegetable salad: Cook quinoa and mix it with crunchy vegetables such as cucumber, peppers, carrots and cherry tomatoes. Dress with olive oil and lemon juice.

5. Lentil and vegetable soup: Prepare a comforting soup with cooked lentils, carrots, celery, onion and low-sodium vegetable broth. Add spices such as turmeric and cumin for flavor.

6. Turkey and avocado wrap: Wrap slices of low-salt turkey and avocado in a whole wheat tortilla. Add lettuce, tomato and cucumber for extra fiber and texture.

7. Chickpea and vegetable salad: Combine cooked chickpeas, cucumber, tomato, peppers and onion in a salad bowl. Dress with olive oil, lemon juice, and a pinch of salt and pepper.

8. Salmon and avocado wrap: Wrap grilled salmon in a whole wheat tortilla. Add avocado, spinach and thin cucumber slices. For extra flavor, add a low-fat yogurt sauce.

9. Pumpkin and ginger soup: Cook diced pumpkin in low-sodium vegetable broth and grated fresh ginger. Blend the mixture to a smooth, creamy texture. Garnish with low-fat sour cream and fresh cilantro.

10. Spinach and Salmon Salad: Combine fresh spinach with grilled salmon chunks, cherry tomatoes, cucumber and walnuts. Dress with olive oil, lemon juice, and a pinch of salt.

11. Chicken and Vegetable Wraps: Wrap grilled chicken breasts in a whole wheat tortilla. Add bell pepper strips, shredded carrots and lettuce leaves. Serve with a low-fat dip, such as herbed Greek yogurt.

12. Vegetable soup: Prepare a comforting soup with low-sodium vegetable broth and add carrots, zucchini and peppers. Add herbs such as parsley and thyme for flavor.

13. Quinoa and vegetable salad: Cook quinoa and mix it with crunchy vegetables such as cucumber, peppers, carrots and cherry tomatoes. Dress with olive oil and lemon juice.

14. Baked turkey with mashed sweet potatoes: Season a breast with herbs and spices before baking. Serve with mashed sweet potatoes made with roasted sweet potatoes, a little low-fat milk, and a pinch of cinnamon.

15. Tofu and vegetable stir-fry: Sauté cubed tofu with various vegetables such as broccoli, carrots, bell peppers and mushrooms. Add low-sodium soy sauce and serve with brown rice.

16. Baked fish with vegetables: Bake a portion of white fish, such as sole or hake, with lemon, pepper and herbs of your choice. Serve with various roasted vegetables, such as carrots, broccoli and zucchini.

17. Grilled chicken salad: Combine chicken chunks with lettuce leaves, cherry tomatoes, cucumber, avocado and walnuts. Dress with a light lemon and olive oil vinaigrette.

18. Whole wheat pasta with homemade tomato sauce: Cook whole wheat pasta al dente and accompany it with a homemade tomato sauce made with fresh tomatoes, onion, garlic, and herbs such as basil and oregano. Add vegetables such as spinach or sautéed mushrooms.

19. Chickpea and avocado salad: Combine cooked chickpeas, diced avocado, cucumber, tomato, red onion and fresh cilantro. Dress with lemon juice, olive oil, salt and pepper.

20. Shrimp and vegetable stir-fry: Sauté shrimp with peppers, carrots, broccoli, and onion in olive oil in a skillet. Add low-sodium soy sauce and serve with brown rice.

21. Quinoa and smoked salmon salad: Combine cooked quinoa, diced smoked salmon, spinach, cherry tomatoes and avocado in a salad bowl. Dress with a lemon vinaigrette and Dijon mustard.

22. Quinoa and roasted vegetable salad: Cook quinoa and mix it with roasted vegetables such as squash, eggplant, carrots and peppers. Dress with olive oil, balsamic vinegar, and a pinch of salt and pepper.

23. Chicken curry with brown rice: Grill chicken in a homemade sauce made with coconut milk, red curry paste, garlic and ginger. Serve with brown rice.

24. Tuna and avocado wrap: Combine canned tuna, water, and avocado in a whole wheat tortilla. Add spinach leaves, sliced tomato, and a low-fat salsa of your choice.

25. Pumpkin and ginger soup: Cook diced pumpkin in low-sodium vegetable broth and grated fresh ginger. Blend the mixture to a smooth, creamy texture. Garnish with low-fat sour cream and fresh cilantro.

26. Lentil and vegetable salad: Combine cooked lentils with cucumber, peppers, red onion and fresh parsley. Dress with lemon juice, olive oil, salt and pepper.

27. Baked turkey with cauliflower puree: Bake a breast seasoned with herbs and spices. Serve with cauliflower puree made with cooked and mashed cauliflower, a little low-fat milk, and a pinch of nutmeg.

Remember to tailor these recipes to your personal preferences and dietary requirements. Additionally, it is essential to stay well-hydrated by drinking plenty of water throughout the day and to maintain a fiber-rich, balanced diet to prevent constipation, which can often worsen hemorrhoids.

Snacks

1. Greek yogurt with flax seeds: Greek yogurt is rich in protein and an excellent source of fiber. Combine it with flax seeds for a satiating and nutritious snack.

2. Celery sticks with hummus: Celery is low in calories and fiber. Serve it with hummus for added flavor and protein.

3. Fruit and Vegetable Smoothie: Blend spinach, pineapple, cucumber and coconut water into a refreshing and nutritious smoothie. Fruits and vegetables add fiber and essential vitamins.

4. Lettuce wraps: Wrap grilled chicken strips, avocado and lettuce leaves in a roll. Add hummus or Greek yogurt dip as a topping.

5. Kale chips: Bake kale leaves with olive oil and salt until crispy. These kale chips are rich in fiber and nutrients.

6. Fruit smoothie with yogurt: Blend your favorite fruits, such as berries or melon, with unsweetened yogurt and ice. Add ground flax seeds for a fiber boost.

7. Fruit bowl with nuts: Prepare a bowl with fresh fruits, such as kiwi, pineapple and grapes, and add a handful of nuts. Nuts provide healthy fats and fiber.

8. Ham and cucumber rolls: Wrap slices of lean ham around cucumber slices. For extra flavor, add a thin layer of fat-free cream cheese.

9. Yogurt with homemade granola: Choose plain, unsweetened yogurt and add granola with oats, nuts and seeds.

Granola provides fiber and a crunchy texture.

Dinner Ideas

1. Baked fish with roasted vegetables: Bake a portion of white fish, such as salmon or hake, with lemon, pepper and herbs of your choice. Serve with various roasted vegetables, such as squash, carrots and broccoli.

2. Grilled chicken salad: Combine chicken chunks with spinach leaves, cherry tomatoes, cucumber, avocado and walnuts. Dress with a light lemon and olive oil vinaigrette.

3. Vegetable soup: Prepare a comforting soup with low-sodium vegetable broth and add carrots, broccoli and peppers. Add herbs such as parsley and thyme for flavor.

4. Chickpea and avocado salad: Combine cooked chickpeas, diced avocado, cucumber, tomato, red onion and fresh cilantro. Dress with lemon juice, olive oil, salt and pepper.

5. Shrimp and vegetable stir-fry: Sauté shrimp with peppers, carrots, broccoli, and onion in olive oil in a skillet. Add low-sodium soy sauce and serve with brown rice.

6. Quinoa and smoked salmon salad: Combine cooked quinoa, smoked salmon chunks, spinach, cherry tomatoes and avocado in a salad bowl. Dress with a lemon Dijon mustard vinaigrette.

7. Baked chicken with cauliflower puree: Season a chicken breast with herbs and spices before baking. Serve with cauliflower puree made with cooked and mashed cauliflower, a little low-fat milk, and a pinch of nutmeg.

8. Spinach and Salmon Salad: Combine fresh spinach with grilled salmon chunks, cherry tomatoes, cucumber and walnuts. Dress with olive oil, lemon juice, and a pinch of salt.

9. Turkey and avocado wrap: Wrap a slice of low-sodium turkey and avocado in a whole wheat tortilla. Add lettuce leaves, sliced tomato, and a low-fat salsa of your choice.

10. Lentil soup: Cook lentils in low-sodium vegetable broth with onion, carrots and celery. Add herbs such as thyme and rosemary for flavor.

11. Tofu and vegetable stir-fry: Stir-fry cubed tofu with broccoli, carrots, bell peppers and mushrooms. Add low-sodium soy sauce and serve with brown rice noodles.

12. Quinoa and vegetable salad: Cook quinoa and mix it with crunchy vegetables such as cucumber, peppers, carrots and cherry tomatoes. Dress with olive oil and lemon juice.

13. Grilled fish with sautéed spinach: Grill fish, such as salmon or sea bass, and serve with spinach sautéed in olive oil and garlic.

14. Grilled chicken and quinoa salad: Combine grilled chicken chunks with cooked quinoa, cherry tomatoes, cucumber, red onion and lettuce leaves. Dress with a light lemon and olive oil vinaigrette.

15. Pumpkin soup with ginger: Cook diced pumpkin in low-sodium vegetable broth and grated fresh ginger. Blend the mixture to a smooth, creamy texture. Garnish with low-fat sour cream and fresh cilantro.

16. Chickpea and avocado salad: Combine cooked chickpeas, diced avocado, tomato, cucumber, red onion and fresh cilantro. Dress with lemon juice, olive oil, salt and pepper.

17. Shrimp and vegetable stir-fry: Sauté shrimp with peppers, carrots, broccoli, and onion in a skillet with olive oil. Add low-sodium soy sauce and serve with brown rice.

18. Quinoa and smoked salmon salad: Combine cooked quinoa, diced smoked salmon, spinach, cherry tomatoes and avocado in a salad bowl. Dress with a lemon vinaigrette and Dijon mustard.

19. Baked chicken with steamed vegetables: Bake a chicken breast seasoned with herbs and spices, accompanied with various steamed vegetables such as broccoli, carrots and cauliflower.

20. Salmon and avocado salad: Combine grilled salmon chunks with diced avocado, spinach, cherry tomatoes and walnuts. Dress with a light lemon and olive oil vinaigrette.

21. Vegetable and lentil soup: Prepare a comforting soup with low-sodium vegetable broth. Add carrots, celery, peppers and lentils. For flavor, add herbs such as parsley and thyme.

22. Chickpea and spinach salad: Combine cooked chickpeas, fresh spinach, cherry tomatoes, cucumber and olives. Dress with olive oil, lemon juice, and a pinch of salt.

23. Tofu and vegetable stir-fry with brown rice: Sauté cubed tofu with a variety of vegetables, such as peppers, carrots, broccoli and mushrooms, in a skillet with olive oil. Add low-sodium soy sauce and serve with brown rice.

JUICES AND SMOOTHIES

"Enjoy your good health; only those who are well are young"
(Voltaire)

Raw foods, often referred to as "living" foods, are an exceptional source of vitamins, minerals, fiber, trace elements, enzymes, and other vital compounds that support overall health. Incorporating these nutrient-rich foods into your daily diet not only aids in disease prevention but also alleviates symptoms of various health conditions, slows down the aging process, balances gut flora, and enhances energy levels and vitality.

While salads, whole fruits, and nuts are excellent raw food options, one of the easiest and most convenient ways to ensure regular intake is by preparing homemade juices, smoothies, and shakes. These beverages serve as a delicious and practical alternative for individuals who may not enjoy consuming fruits and vegetables directly, making it easier to include these essential nutrients in their diet.

In today's world, where ultra-processed foods and toxins have become increasingly prevalent, the need for natural, nutrient-dense foods is more crucial than ever. Raw foods play a vital role in supporting detoxification, maintaining health, and restoring balance to the body.

Many people tend to prepare their juices and smoothies using only fruits, often overlooking the incredible health benefits vegetables and leafy greens provide. Adding these to your recipes not only increases variety but also significantly boosts their nutritional value, enhancing their antioxidant, remineralizing, toning, and alkalizing properties. These qualities help maintain the body's balance, rejuvenate cells, and promote overall well-being. Additionally, vegetables and greens lower the glycemic index, improve satiety, and maximize the health benefits of these preparations.

However, it is crucial to understand that most store-bought juices are far from healthy options. These commercial products are often loaded with excessive added sugars, artificial sweeteners, preservatives, and harmful chemical additives.

Furthermore, the pasteurization processes used during production strip away essential vitamins and enzymes, rendering them nutritionally deficient. The high level of refinement also removes fiber, a vital component of whole foods. In many cases, these juices contain only minimal amounts of actual fruit, making them highly processed and lacking true nutritional value.

One major concern with many juices and smoothies is their high glycemic index, which can cause blood sugar spikes, lead to weight gain, and contribute to long-term metabolic imbalances. To truly enjoy healthy and nourishing beverages, the best approach is to prepare them at home using fresh, natural, and high-quality ingredients. Homemade juices and smoothies are packed with nutrients that provide genuine benefits for your body and overall well-being.

Incorporating fresh juices made from fruits, vegetables, and leafy greens into your daily routine is an excellent practice for maintaining a healthy and energetic body. With endless combinations to explore, you can enjoy not only flavorful and refreshing options but also targeted health benefits, such as relief from conditions like arthritis, thanks to essential nutrients that support wellness. Making this a part of your everyday life can transform your health, boost your energy, and elevate your quality of life. Try it for yourself and feel the difference!

Benefits for Hemorrhoids

Juices, smoothies, and shakes are not only delicious and refreshing but can also serve as powerful allies in alleviating hemorrhoid symptoms and promoting recovery. Their high content of fiber, antioxidants, and water makes these beverages a valuable aid in improving intestinal health and enhancing overall well-being. Here are their primary benefits:

‣ **Optimal Hydration**: Drinking juices, smoothies, and shakes helps keep the body well-hydrated, which is essential to preventing constipation–one of the main causes of hemorrhoids. Adequate hydration softens stools, making them easier to pass and reducing strain during bowel movements.

‣ **High Fiber Content**: When smoothies are prepared with whole fruits and vegetables, their fiber content is preserved. Fiber is a vital nutrient for regulating bowel movements, preventing constipation, and reducing pressure on the veins in the rectum and anus.

‣ **Anti-inflammatory and Soothing Properties**: Many commonly used ingredients in juices and smoothies, such as blueberries, pineapple, ginger, and turmeric, contain anti-inflammatory properties that can help reduce hemorrhoid-related inflammation, relieving pain and discomfort.

‣ **Digestive Support**: Fresh combinations of fruits and vegetables support efficient digestion, helping to maintain a healthy digestive system. Ingredients like papaya, pineapple, and green apple are particularly effective in aiding digestion and preventing intestinal complications.

‣ **Quick Nutrient Absorption**: Juices and smoothies allow for the rapid absorption of essential nutrients, including vitamins, minerals, and antioxidants. These nutrients play a crucial role in strengthening the immune system and accelerating the healing of damaged tissues.

‣ **Support for a Light Diet**: These beverages provide a convenient and versatile option for maintaining a light, balanced diet. As they are easy to digest, they minimize irritation to the gastrointestinal system–an especially important benefit for those dealing with painful hemorrhoids.

Star Ingredients to Fight Hemorrhoids

Boost the benefits of your recipes by including these valuable ingredients:

‣ *Plums and Pears*: Rich in soluble fiber, these fruits are ideal for promoting healthy bowel movements.

‣ *Papaya and Pineapple*: Known for their natural enzymes, which help improve digestion.

‣ *Spinach and Kale*: Loaded with iron, fiber, and antioxidants for overall health benefits.

‣ *Blueberries and Raspberries*: Exceptional antioxidants with powerful anti-inflammatory properties.

‣ *Ginger and Turmeric*: Great for improving circulation and reducing inflammation.

Adding juices, smoothies, and shakes to your diet is not only a delicious choice but also an effective way to relieve and prevent hemorrhoids. At the same time, you'll enjoy a healthy, nutritious, and satisfying way of eating. Your gut health will thank you!

General Health Benefits

Including smoothies or shakes in your diet is an excellent choice for improving your overall health. Here are some of their most notable benefits:

▸ **Compliance with Recommended Fruit and Vegetable Intake:** Smoothies and shakes offer a practical and enjoyable way to meet the daily recommendation of five servings of fruits and vegetables. They provide a diverse range of essential nutrients that support optimal health and overall well-being.

▸ **Easy Assimilation and Digestion:** As liquid meals, smoothies and shakes are gentler on the digestive system and allow for quicker nutrient absorption. They are especially beneficial for individuals with digestive sensitivities or challenges.

▸ **Vitamin and Mineral Powerhouse:** Made from fresh fruits and vegetables, smoothies and shakes are rich sources of essential vitamins and minerals that promote the proper functioning of the body.

▸ **Detoxification and Cleansing:** Ingredients like leafy greens and natural antioxidants help flush out toxins, enhance cell health, and support effective internal cleansing.

▸ **Balancing Body pH:** By incorporating alkaline foods, smoothies and shakes play a key role in stabilizing the body's pH levels, aiding disease prevention and improving overall wellness.

▸ **Reduction of Inflammation:** Anti-inflammatory additions such as turmeric, ginger, and leafy greens can help minimize inflammation, fostering better health and increased comfort.

▸ **A Balanced Meal Replacement:** When combined with protein, healthy fats, and complex carbohydrates, smoothies become a nourishing and balanced meal replacement. They provide sustained energy and promote fullness throughout the day.

▸ **Supports Weight Management:** With their low-calorie yet nutrient-dense profiles, smoothies and shakes encourage healthy eating habits. They help manage appetite and support maintaining or achieving an ideal weight.

▸ **Enhances Skin Health**: Packed with skin-friendly vitamins like A and C from fresh ingredients, smoothies and shakes contribute to hydrated, radiant, and healthy skin.

▸ **Slows Cellular Aging**: The antioxidants in smoothie ingredients combat oxidative damage, protect cells, and help maintain a youthful appearance.

▸ **Boosts Energy and Vitality**: Smoothies made with superfoods provide a steady energy boost, helping you stay active, energized, and revitalized throughout the day.

In conclusion, smoothies and shakes are a nutritious, convenient, and versatile addition to your diet. Not only do they simplify meeting your daily fruit and vegetable intake, but they also provide a wide range of benefits for your overall health and well-being–all in a delicious and effortless way to enjoy.

Homemade vs. Commercial Juices

Nowadays, identifying which foods truly benefit our health can be quite challenging. Supermarkets are overflowing with an extensive range of options, flaunting attractive packaging and clever designs that promise to be natural and healthy. While advertising and packaging often catch our attention, are we genuinely purchasing natural beverages made from fruits and vegetables? Do you know the key differences between homemade juices and industrial products? Are packaged products really as nutritious as they claim to be? Taking a few moments to carefully read ingredient labels and analyze their composition may uncover some surprising truths.

A few years ago, international regulations were established to define the standards that every fruit-based beverage must meet, specifying precise characteristics for each type of product. Below, we'll explore these distinctions and delve into the essential differences.

▸ **Fruit Juice**
Fruit juice is derived from fresh, chilled, or frozen fruits without undergoing any fermentation. It may contain separately extracted pulp and, in some cases, be blended with juice from various fruits. Labels are required to specify the composition in descending order, including the exact percentage of each fruit.

To prolong shelf life and eliminate the need for refrigeration, fruit juice is typically sterilized or pasteurized. Unfortunately, these processes result in significant nutrient loss, particularly impacting essential vitamins and enzymes. Moreover, the juice lacks the natural fiber found in whole fruits.

‣ Juice from Concentrates
Juice from concentrates is created by reconstituting dehydrated juice concentrates with water. Concentrates are produced by extracting natural juice through evaporation or other physical methods. During reconstitution, manufacturers may add aromas or pulp from similar fruits to partially restore flavor.

Though widely consumed, these juices suffer nutrient losses during production, including enzymes, vitamins, minerals, and the valuable fiber that characterizes natural fruit.

‣ Dehydrated or Powdered Fruit Juice
This product is manufactured by removing water from fruit to create a dry powder, which can later be rehydrated or sold in its dehydrated state. However, the dehydration process significantly diminishes its nutritional value, leading to the loss of enzymes, vitamins, minerals, and natural fiber.

‣ Fruit Nectar
Fruit nectar differs from pure juice as it is made using fruit concentrate, water, and added sugars or sweeteners. Its nutritional value is considerably lower compared to natural fruit juices due to its inclusion of artificial additives to enhance flavor, color, or shelf life.

‣ Juice-Based Drinks
These beverages typically combine various fruits but contain minimal actual fruit juice. Often, they lack the essential nutrients derived from fruits, consisting largely of water, artificial aromas, colorings, and sweeteners.

‣ Milk-Infused Juice Drinks
Milk-infused juice drinks include fruit juice, often from concentrates, in very small proportions. They are mixed with milk, water, flavorings, and other ingredients. These beverages are not considered true juices, and any nutrients present are artificially added during manufacturing to compensate for losses incurred during processing.

‣ Vegetable and/or Greens Juice
Vegetable and greens juices are extracted from vegetables using specialized industrial methods, often with added pulp or pureed

ingredients. They may also blend various vegetables to create balanced or palatable flavors.

To extend shelf life and eliminate refrigeration requirements, these juices undergo pasteurization or sterilization, which unfortunately reduces essential nutrients, including vitamins and phytonutrients. Additionally, they lack the natural fiber of whole vegetables and may include preservatives, salt, or flavor enhancers that compromise their nutritional profile.

▸ **Commercial Smoothies**
Commercial smoothies are typically prepared by blending fruits, vegetables, and greens–often using purees or concentrates –with water, milk, plant-based beverages, or similar liquids. Their thicker texture comes from a higher proportion of pulp or fiber-rich components.

To enhance taste, appearance, and shelf life, industrial smoothies usually contain added sugars, preservatives, colorings, and flavorings that alter their natural composition. Moreover, they undergo pasteurization or thermal sterilization to allow room-temperature storage, further degrading their original nutrients and reducing their overall nutritional quality.

Advantages of Homemade Juices
After discovering what commercial products truly contain, it becomes evident that making juices at home offers numerous advantages. Here are the key benefits:

▸ **Complete Control Over Ingredients**: Preparing your own juices allows you to ensure the quality of the ingredients you use. There are no unnecessary additives, no preservatives, and –most importantly–no unpleasant surprises.

▸ **Variety and Creativity**: You have the freedom to choose your favorite fruits and vegetables, experiment with unique combinations, or incorporate fresh, seasonal produce. This not only provides a burst of delicious flavors but also boosts your intake of essential nutrients.

▸ **Authentic Aroma and Flavor**: Homemade juices retain the genuine aroma and taste of fresh fruits and vegetables. There's truly nothing like enjoying a freshly made juice packed with natural freshness.

▸ **Maximum Nutrient Retention**: Vitamins, minerals, enzymes, antioxidants, and other nutrients remain intact when you prepare juices at home, significantly enhancing their health benefits.

▶ **Premium Quality Ingredients**: Choosing fresh, seasonal produce at its peak ripeness ensures optimal flavor and exceptional nutritional value.

▶ **Seasonal Food Benefits**: Consuming fruits and vegetables that are in season supports sustainability, is more cost-effective, and often results in better taste and nutritional quality.

▶ **Total Customization**: Whether using a juicer or blender, you can adjust the consistency of your juice to your liking– whether you prefer a light, clear juice or a thicker, fiber-rich option.

▶ **Kid-Friendly Option**: Homemade juices are an excellent way to incorporate fruits and vegetables into children's diets, especially for picky eaters. With creative flavors and fun presentations, you can make juices irresistible for kids.

Making juices at home provides several compelling advantages: complete control over ingredients, enhanced nutrient retention, and the flexibility to tailor your drinks to your preferences. It's also a simple yet effective way to promote healthy eating for the whole family.

Possible Adverse Effects

If you suffer from **constipation, gastritis, colitis, irritable bowel syndrome, or SIBO**, it's essential to take certain precautions when preparing smoothies or juices. Following these recommendations will help you enjoy their benefits without worsening your symptoms:

▶ **Use a juicer instead of a blender**: For digestive health conditions, it's often better to use a juicer rather than a blender when making juices. Juicing removes most of the fiber from the ingredients, resulting in a smoother liquid that is gentler on your digestive system.

▶ **Moderate your fiber intake**: Although fiber is highly beneficial for overall health, excessive consumption can lead to gas, bloating, or constipation–especially for individuals with sensitive digestion. Be mindful of the fiber content in your smoothies by limiting ingredients like fruit pulp, seeds, and whole grains.

‣ **Introduce juices gradually**: If you're unsure how your body will react, start with small portions. This enables you to monitor their effects on your digestion and adjust the recipes to suit your specific needs.

‣ **Consume juices on an empty stomach**: Drinking juices on an empty stomach can maximize nutrient absorption and aid digestion. This approach minimizes the risk of digestive discomfort and helps you fully benefit from the juice's nutrients

‣ **Tailor recipes to your personal needs**: Everyone's digestive system is unique, and responses to certain foods can vary greatly. Pay close attention to how your body reacts after consuming juices, and adapt ingredient combinations to best support your health and well-being.

The best time to have them

There are several effective ways to incorporate juices into your routine, depending on your goals and daily habits. Below are three recommended methods:

‣ **In the morning, on an empty stomach**: Begin your day with a carefully chosen juice recipe, consuming it before eating anything else. Drinking juice on an empty stomach enhances nutrient absorption and stimulates your digestive system, helping prepare it for the rest of the day.

‣ **On an empty stomach, before meals**: Enjoy a juice approximately 30 minutes before your main meals to maximize its benefits. This practice supports digestion and boosts nutrient absorption, promoting overall health and well-being.

‣ **Juice-based fasting**: Engage in a multi-day fast consisting exclusively of juices to achieve specific health objectives or to detoxify your body. Choose 2 to 3 recipes and consume them consistently throughout the day to stay nourished and energized.

Preparation Tips

Preparing fresh juices is an easy and nutritious way to make the most of the vitamins and minerals found in fruits and vegetables. To optimize the process and ensure safety, consider the following recommendations:

‣ **Choose organic ingredients**: Whenever possible, opt for organic fruits and vegetables. They provide cleaner, pesticide-free consumption and promote a healthier lifestyle.

▸ **Wash ingredients thoroughly**: Rinse all produce carefully to remove dirt, bacteria, and chemical residues. Trim any bruised, moldy, or damaged areas to prevent contamination.

▸ **Cut ingredients into smaller pieces**: Make blending easier by chopping fruits and vegetables into smaller, manageable chunks. This helps achieve a smoother texture and shortens preparation time.

▸ **Balance ingredients with low water content**: Fruits and vegetables with low water content, such as bananas and avocados, may require pre-mixing. Start with juicier ingredients to create a liquid base, then gradually add denser items for a cohesive blend.

▸ **Peel certain fruits appropriately**: Remove citrus rinds (like those from oranges and grapefruits), as their outer layers may contain toxins. However, keep the nutrient-rich white inner layer. Peel tropical fruits, such as papayas and kiwis, especially if they are grown in regions with less stringent chemical regulations.

▸ **Discard harmful seeds**: Remove seeds from apples, as they contain trace amounts of cyanide and are unsafe to consume. On the other hand, seeds from grapes, melons, lemons, and limes are safe and offer additional health benefits.

▸ **Incorporate stems and leaves mindfully**: Many stems and leaves are nutritious, but be cautious. Avoid toxic ones, such as carrot and rhubarb leaves, which can be harmful.

▸ **Drink your juice immediately**: Freshly prepared juice is best consumed right away to minimize nutrient loss and avoid oxidation. This ensures maximum freshness and health benefits.

▸ **Remove bitter celery leaves**: Bitter celery leaves can affect the flavor of your juice. Remove them before blending the stalks to create a more balanced and enjoyable taste.

Key Recommendations

Smoothies and shakes are an excellent, healthy alternative, but to get the most out of them, it's essential to keep certain aspects in mind. Below are some key recommendations:

▸ **Moderate fruit consumption:** Fruits are a fantastic source of nutrients but also contain fructose, a natural sugar that, when consumed excessively, can impact your health. Strive for balance by moderating your fruit intake throughout the day. Additionally, avoid eating fruits at night, as the body may metabolize them less efficiently during this time.

▸ **Choose seasonal fruits:** Seasonal fruits are often more nutrient-rich, flavorful, and cost-effective. By opting for fruits in season, you can enjoy their peak freshness and nutritional benefits while saving money.

▸ **Pick compatible combinations:** Not all fruits or ingredients blend well together. Research suitable pairings to create a smoothie or shake with balanced flavors and optimal nutritional value.

▸ **Use a moderate amount of ingredients:** The simplest smoothies are often the best. Avoid overloading them with excessive ingredients, which can lead to heavy textures or digestive discomfort. Stick to recommended recipes and be mindful of proportions.

▸ **Include leafy greens and vegetables:** Incorporate leafy greens, like spinach or kale, or vegetables, such as cucumber, to lower the glycemic index and boost your drink's nutrient profile. These additions make your smoothie both healthier and more satisfying.

▸ **Use natural sweeteners in moderation:** Enjoy the natural flavors of the ingredients, but if sweetening is necessary, choose options like raw honey or pure stevia. Use them sparingly to maintain a balanced nutritional profile.

▸ **Chew your drink:** Even liquid smoothies benefit from being "chewed." This simple habit stimulates the release of digestive enzymes, helping improve nutrient absorption and reducing discomfort like bloating or indigestion.

▸ **Store properly:** For the best results, consume smoothies or shakes fresh. If storing is needed, place them in a dark, airtight container in the refrigerator, or freeze individual portions for later use.

▸ **Make them fun and personalized:** Add an enjoyable twist by freezing smoothies in molds with fun shapes–an excellent way to turn a healthy drink into a delightful treat, especially for children.

These recommendations will help you make the most of your smoothies and shakes. While the recipes provided in this book are crafted to facilitate nutrient absorption, always remember that individual needs vary. Feel free to experiment with different combinations, tailor recipes to suit your tastes, and prioritize your health and well-being. Enjoy the journey to a healthier lifestyle!

Suggested Recipes

Here's a selection of juices and smoothies specially crafted to help ease the symptoms of hemorrhoids. These recipes, rich in fiber, antioxidants, and essential nutrients, will not only support your intestinal health but also let you enjoy fresh and delicious flavors while taking care of your well-being. Give them a try and feel the difference!

▸ **Pineapple, apple, carrot and cucumber juice:**
Ingredients:
- 1 cup fresh pineapple
- 1 green apple
- 1 large carrot
- 1 cucumber
- 1 kale leaf (optional)
- 1 tablespoon grated fresh ginger
- Juice of half a lemon

Instructions:
1. Prepare all the ingredients and put them through a juicer or blender.
2. Using a blender, strain the juice to remove solid residue.
3. Serve the juice immediately and drink it to get the best benefits.

Benefits:
- Pineapple contains enzymes that reduce inflammation and promote healthy digestion.
- Green apples are fiber-rich, which can help prevent constipation, a common trigger for hemorrhoids.
- Carrots and cucumbers are moisturizing and fiber-rich foods that help keep stools soft and facilitate bowel movements.
- Ginger has anti-inflammatory properties and helps relieve the discomfort associated with hemorrhoids.

- Lemon provides vitamin C, which helps maintain a healthy immune system and improve blood vessel health.

▸ **Beet, carrot and apple juice:**
Ingredients:
- 1 medium beet
- 2 large carrots
- 1 green apple
- Juice of half a lemon
- 1 tablespoon grated fresh ginger

Instructions:
1. Wash and prepare all the ingredients.
2. Run the beets, carrots and green apple through a juicer or blender.
3. Add the lemon juice and grated ginger to the juice.
4. Mix all ingredients well.
5. Serve and drink the juice immediately.

Benefits:
- Beets are rich in antioxidants and help improve blood circulation, which relieves symptoms.
- Carrots contain fiber and vitamin A, which help regulate intestinal transit and promote healthy digestion.
- Green apples are also rich in fiber and can help prevent constipation.
- Ginger has anti-inflammatory properties and helps reduce inflammation and discomfort.
- Lemons provide vitamin C and help strengthen the immune system.

▸ **Watermelon, pineapple, and cucumber juice:**
Ingredients:
- 1 cup watermelon chunks
- 1 cup fresh pineapple chunks
- 1 cucumber
- 1 tablespoon chia seeds
- Juice of half a lemon

Instructions:
1. Wash and prepare all the ingredients.
2. Run the watermelon, pineapple and cucumber through a juicer or blender.
3. Add the lemon juice and chia seeds to the juice.
4. Mix all ingredients well.
5. Serve and drink the juice immediately.

Benefits:
- Watermelon is rich in water and helps hydrate and soften the stool, facilitating bowel movements and relieving discomfort.
- Pineapple contains bromelain, an enzyme that helps reduce inflammation and promote healthy digestion.
- Cucumbers are moisturizing and rich in fiber, which can help keep stools soft and prevent constipation.
- Chia seeds are an excellent source of fiber and help regulate intestinal transit.
- Lemons provide vitamin C and help strengthen the immune system.

‣ **Carrot, apple, and parsley juice:**
Ingredients:
- 2 large carrots
- 1 green apple
- A handful of fresh parsley leaves
- Juice of half a lemon

Instructions:
1. Wash and prepare all the ingredients.
2. Pass the carrots, green apple and parsley through a juicer or blender.
3. Add the lemon juice to the juice obtained.
4. Mix all ingredients well.
5. Serve and drink the juice immediately.

Benefits:
- Carrots: They are rich in fiber, which helps promote healthy digestion and prevent constipation.
- Green apple: It contains soluble fiber, which can help soften stools and facilitate evacuation, relieving discomfort.
- Parsley: It has anti-inflammatory and antioxidant properties, which can help reduce inflammation and discomfort caused by hemorrhoids.
- Lemon juice provides vitamin C, strengthening the immune system, and can help improve blood vessel health.

‣ **Carrot and spinach juice:**
Ingredients:
- 2 large carrots
- A handful of fresh spinach
- Juice of half a lemon

Instructions:
1. Wash and prepare all the ingredients.

2. Put the carrots and spinach through a juicer or blender.
3. Add the lemon juice to the juice obtained.
4. Mix all ingredients well.
5. Serve and drink the juice immediately.

Benefits:
- Carrots: They are rich in fiber, which helps promote healthy digestion and prevent constipation, one of the triggers of hemorrhoids.
- Spinach: It contains fiber and nutrients such as magnesium, which help maintain a healthy digestive system and prevent constipation.
- Lemon juice provides vitamin C, strengthening the immune system, and helps improve blood vessel health.

▸ **Celery, apple, carrot and spinach juice:**
Ingredients:
- 2 stalks of celery
- 1 green apple
- 1 large carrot
- A handful of fresh spinach
- Juice of half a lemon

Instructions:
1. Wash and prepare all the ingredients.
2. Run the celery, green apple, carrot and spinach through a juicer or blender.
3. Add the lemon juice to the juice obtained.
4. Mix all ingredients well.
5. Serve and drink the juice immediately.

Benefits:
- Celery contains fiber and water, which help soften the stool and facilitate evacuation, relieving discomfort.
- Green apple: It contains soluble fiber, which helps soften stools and promote healthy digestion.
- Carrot: Helps promote healthy digestion and prevent constipation.
- Spinach: It contains fiber and nutrients such as magnesium, which help maintain a healthy digestive system and prevent constipation.
- Lemon juice: It provides vitamin C, strengthens the immune system, and helps improve blood vessel health.

▸ **Cherry, apple, and carrot juice:**
Ingredients:

- 1 cup fresh cherries (pitted)
- 1 green apple
- 1 large carrot
- 1/2 cup water

Instructions:
1. Wash and pit the cherries.
2. Wash and prepare the green apple and carrot.
3. Pass the cherries, green apple and carrot through a juicer or blender.
4. Add the water to the juice obtained and mix well.
5. Serve and drink the juice immediately.

Benefits:
- Cherries: They are rich in antioxidants and anti-inflammatory compounds, which help reduce inflammation and discomfort.
- Green apple: It contains soluble fiber, which helps soften stools and promote healthy digestion.
- Carrot: It is rich in fiber, which helps promote healthy digestion and prevent constipation.
- Water: Staying hydrated is essential to avoid constipation and keep stools soft.

‣ **Cherry juice:**
Ingredients:
- 1 cup fresh or frozen cherries
- 1 cup of water
- 1 tablespoon lemon juice
- 1 tablespoon honey (optional)

Instructions:
1. Wash the cherries and remove the stems.
2. Place the cherries in a blender with the water, lemon juice and honey (if you want to add a little sweetness).
3. Blend all ingredients until smooth and homogeneous.
4. If you prefer a more liquid consistency, add more water and mix again.

Benefits:
- Cherries are rich in antioxidants and anti-inflammatory compounds that help reduce inflammation and discomfort.
- Vitamin C present in cherries strengthens blood vessels and promotes better circulation.
- The natural fiber in cherries helps regulate intestinal transit and prevent constipation.

‣ **Apple, pear, and ginger juice:**

Ingredients:
- 1 apple
- 1 pear
- 1 small piece of fresh ginger
- 1 cup of water

Instructions:
1. Wash the apple and pear and cut them into small pieces, removing the seeds and core from the apple.
2. Peel the ginger and cut it into small pieces.
3. Place the apple, pear and ginger in a blender along with the water.
4. Blend all ingredients until smooth and homogeneous.

Benefits:
- Apples and pears are rich in fiber, which helps to improve intestinal regularity and prevent constipation.
- Ginger has anti-inflammatory properties and helps reduce inflammation and discomfort.
- The combination of apple, pear and ginger promotes healthy digestion and relieves gastrointestinal symptoms, which is beneficial for people with hemorrhoids.

▸ Juice of carrots, apple, ginger and parsley:
Ingredients:
- 2 carrots
- 1 apple
- 1 small piece of fresh ginger
- A handful of fresh parsley
- 1 cup of water

Instructions:
1. Wash the carrots, apple and parsley.
2. Peel the carrots and cut them into pieces.
3. Cut the apple into chunks, removing the seeds and core.
4. Peel the ginger and cut it into small pieces.
5. Place the carrots, apple, ginger and parsley in a blender with the water.
6. Blend all ingredients until smooth and homogeneous.

Benefits:
- Carrots help regulate intestinal transit, thus reducing the risk of constipation.
- Apples help to improve intestinal regularity.
- Ginger has anti-inflammatory properties and helps reduce inflammation and discomfort.
- Parsley helps strengthen blood vessels and improve blood

circulation.

▶ **Carrot, celery, spinach and parsley juice:**
Ingredients:
- 2 carrots
- 2 stalks of celery
- A handful of fresh spinach
- A handful of fresh parsley
- 1 cup of water

Instructions:
1. Wash the carrots, celery, spinach and parsley.
2. Peel the carrots and cut off the ends of the celery.
3. Cut the carrots, celery and parsley into small pieces.
4. Place the carrots, celery, spinach and parsley in a blender with the water.
5. Blend all ingredients until smooth and homogeneous.

Benefits:
- Carrots help regulate intestinal transit.
- Celery is also a source of fiber and contributes to healthy digestion.
- Spinach is high in fiber and contains antioxidant compounds that help reduce inflammation and discomfort.
- Parsley is rich in nutrients, such as vitamin C and antioxidants, and has anti-inflammatory properties.

▶ **Potato juice, carrots, apple and parsley:**
Ingredients:
- 1 medium potato
- 2 carrots
- 1 apple
- A handful of fresh parsley
- 1 cup of water

Instructions:
1. Wash the potato, carrots, apple and parsley.
2. Peel the potato, carrots and apple.
3. Cut the potato, carrots and apple into small pieces.
4. Place the potato, carrots, apple and parsley in a blender along with the water.
5. Blend all ingredients until smooth and homogeneous.

Benefits:
- Potatoes contain resistant starch and fiber that help improve bowel regularity and prevent constipation.

- Carrots are rich in fiber and contribute to healthy digestion.
- Apple helps to soften the stool and reduce tension during bowel movements.
- Parsley is a source of nutrients and antioxidants and has anti-inflammatory properties.

▸ **Melon juice:**
Ingredients:
- 1 cup of melon cut into small pieces

Instructions:
1. Wash and cut the melon into small pieces.
2. Place the melon chunks in a blender.
3. Blend until smooth and homogeneous.

Benefits:
- Melon is a fruit rich in water and fiber, which helps prevent constipation and aggravates hemorrhoids.
- The high water content of cantaloupe helps keep the stool soft and facilitates its passage during bowel movements.
- In addition, cantaloupe is rich in antioxidants and vitamins, which help strengthen blood vessels and promote better circulation, which is beneficial for people with hemorrhoids.

▸ **Pineapple, apple, and ginger juice:**
Ingredients:
- 1 cup fresh pineapple, cut into chunks
- 1 green apple
- 1 small piece of fresh ginger
- 1 cup of water

Instructions:
1. Wash the pineapple, apple and ginger.
2. Cut the pineapple into chunks.
3. Cut the apple into chunks, removing the seeds and core.
4. Peel the ginger and cut it into small pieces.
5. Place the pineapple, apple and ginger in a blender along with the water.
6. Blend all ingredients until smooth and homogeneous.

Benefits:
- Pineapple is a fruit rich in bromelain, an enzyme that has anti-inflammatory properties and helps reduce inflammation.
- Apples help to improve intestinal regularity.
- Ginger has anti-inflammatory properties and helps relieve inflammation and pain in hemorrhoids.

> **Juice of sweet turnips, pears and apples:**
Ingredients:
- 1 sweet turnip
- 2 ripe pears
- 2 green apples

Instructions:
1. Wash all ingredients thoroughly.
2. Peel the sweet turnip and cut into small pieces.
3. Cut the pears and apples into chunks without removing the skin.
4. Place all ingredients in a blender.
5. Blend until smooth and homogeneous.
6. If you wish, you can strain the juice to remove any solid residue.

Benefits:
- Sweet turnip is known for its fiber content, which helps improve intestinal transit and reduces straining during bowel movements.
- Pears and apples are fruits rich in fiber, water and antioxidants, which help keep the digestive system healthy and regular.

> **Juice of carrots, parsley, celery and garlic:**
Ingredients:
- 4 carrots
- A handful of fresh parsley
- 2 stalks of celery
- 2 cloves of garlic

Instructions:
1. Wash all ingredients thoroughly.
2. Peel the carrots and cut them into pieces.
3. Cut the parsley, celery and garlic into smaller pieces.
4. Place all ingredients in a blender.
5. Blend until smooth and homogeneous.
6. If you wish, you can strain the juice to remove any solid residue.

Benefits:
- Carrots help improve digestion and promote intestinal health.
- Parsley is known for its anti-inflammatory properties and helps reduce inflammation.
- Celery helps to facilitate bowel movements.

- Garlic has anti-inflammatory properties and helps improve blood circulation, which is beneficial for hemorrhoids.

▸ **Cherry, lime, and grape juice:**

Ingredients:
- 1 cup cherries (pitted)
- Juice of 1 lime
- 1 cup grapes (preferably seedless)

Instructions:
1. Wash all ingredients thoroughly.
2. Remove the pits from the cherries if necessary.
3. Squeeze the juice from a lime.
4. Place the cherries, lime juice and grapes in a blender.
5. Blend until smooth and homogeneous.
6. If you wish, you can strain the juice to remove any solid residue.

Benefits:
- Cherries are known for their antioxidant content and anti-inflammatory compounds, which help reduce inflammation.
- Lime is rich in vitamin C, which strengthens blood vessels and improves circulation, which is beneficial for hemorrhoids.
- Grapes contain fiber and antioxidants, which help maintain a healthy digestive system and promote bowel regularity.

MEDICINAL PLANTS

"Investing in health will yield enormous returns"
(Gro Harlem Brundtland)

Since time immemorial, humanity has turned to the natural world for answers to its needs. Medicinal herbs, faithful companions on this journey, have generously shared their wisdom to ease ailments and enhance well-being. This ancient knowledge, carefully preserved through the ages, has found a renewed place in the modern world, offering a healthy and sustainable option to address today's challenges.

In a society increasingly conscious of the adverse effects of certain pharmaceutical treatments and the environmental toll of unsustainable practices, botanical remedies are experiencing a resurgence with renewed prominence. For those seeking a balanced, respectful lifestyle in harmony with the environment, these green treasures provide invaluable solutions. This revival not only reflects a growing interest in ecological approaches but also an evolution toward holistic care for both the body and the planet.

What makes these natural wonders truly extraordinary is the complexity of their compounds, capable of delivering antioxidant, anti-inflammatory, antibacterial, and antiviral properties, among others. Their potential ranges from alleviating everyday issues like sleeplessness or sluggish digestion to addressing conditions such as chronic stress or age-related ailments.

Beyond the ability to target specific concerns, these species serve as vital sources of micronutrients–vitamins, minerals, fiber, and antioxidants–that fortify the immune system and support long-term health. Incorporating them into dietary or self-care routines offers a simple, sustainable, and effective path toward illness prevention and enhanced overall wellness.

The botanical kingdom boasts remarkable diversity, featuring countless species uniquely suited to meet specific needs. Whether prepared as herbal teas, applied as balms or tinctures, or utilized in the form of essential oils, their applications are as versatile as they are effective, seamlessly fitting into various lifestyles.

More than mere remedies, these natural allies inspire us to reconnect with the world around us. Harnessing their benefits requires respect for environmental rhythms and a deeper appreciation for our planet's ecosystems. Each herb or extract serves as a tangible reminder of our connection to the living world, fostering a sense of harmony that transcends the physical and nurtures the spiritual.

In addition to their myriad health benefits, plant-based solutions stand out for their accessibility and practical versatility. Many species grow abundantly in wild habitats or can be easily cultivated in home gardens, offering an affordable, sustainable alternative. In a global context marked by economic inequalities, these wellness allies provide inclusive options to complement–or even replace–costly interventions.

Over the centuries, knowledge of these natural solutions has been carefully preserved through oral traditions and written records. This heritage, rooted in deep respect for biodiversity, has been bolstered by modern science, validating the effects of their active compounds and shedding light on their mechanisms of action. It represents a powerful synergy between tradition and innovation, broadening the therapeutic applications of these botanical marvels.

However, unlocking their full potential requires responsible use. Every human body is unique, and while these species possess well-documented therapeutic properties, they are not without risks. Misuse or interactions with conventional medications can lead to adverse effects. Therefore, obtaining accurate and reliable information is essential to ensure safe and effective usage.

One particularly fascinating aspect is how the components within a plant work in unison. Whole extracts, resulting from this intricate interaction, often produce more balanced and holistic effects compared to isolated compounds. Molecules interact in complementary ways, maximizing benefits while reducing potential side effects. Conversely, isolated active principles can provide concentrated solutions but may carry an increased risk of adverse effects on the body.

The innate harmony of these botanical wonders highlights one of biodiversity's greatest gifts–balance. Whole extracts are celebrated for their gentleness and ability to integrate seamlessly with the body's natural processes. On the other hand, synthesized compounds strive for potency, often at the expense of stability. The synergistic interaction between molecular components amplifies therapeutic benefits while limiting potential downsides, making them a choice deeply aligned with human needs.

Ultimately, medicinal plants transcend their role as therapeutic tools–they bridge ancestral wisdom and scientific innovation. They remind us that the health of our bodies and the well-being of our planet are profoundly interconnected. By safeguarding this invaluable legacy, we nurture not only our own health but also that of future generations, renewing the delicate balance between humanity and nature.

Essential Information
Although plants are natural in origin, they should not be considered entirely harmless. Their active compounds may cause adverse effects or trigger allergies in certain individuals.

Occasional consumption of an infusion is unlikely to cause harm. However, excessive, prolonged, or frequent use may result in discomfort, allergic reactions, or even toxicity.

Tolerance to natural remedies varies greatly among individuals. If you are pregnant, breastfeeding, or managing conditions such as chronic illnesses, allergies, kidney or liver insufficiency, cancer, or undergoing medical treatment, it is crucial to refer to the section titled "**Learn Everything You Need to Know About the Plants**" before using them. This section provides essential information on potential risks, contraindications, and interactions, enabling you to make informed and responsible decisions.

Guidelines for Care with Herbal Remedies
For best results, continue using the remedies until your symptoms have completely disappeared. The treatment duration will vary depending on factors like the severity of your condition, how it progresses, your personal commitment, and other important influences.

Keep in mind that some plants or herbal remedies are not suited for continuous or long-term use. In such cases, you will always find specific instructions that address this.

While following the guidelines for the remedies below, it is just as important to focus on the underlying causes of your symptoms. To better understand the root of your health concerns, I recommend referring to the first chapter of this book, specifically the section titled "Causes," where you'll discover essential insights into tackling the problem at its source.

Finally, remember that patience is vital. A condition that has lingered for months or years cannot be resolved in just a few days. Stay committed, persevere, and always prioritize your health and well-being.

Measurements

To achieve the best results when preparing infusions, decoctions, or other plant-based recipes, it is essential to follow these dosage guidelines:

- A tablespoon refers to a level tablespoon.
- A teaspoon refers to a level teaspoon.

Effective Plants for External Use

The topical application of medicinal plants can be highly effective in alleviating the symptoms of hemorrhoids. Depending on the severity of your discomfort, combining them with internal remedies is recommended for faster and more comprehensive relief. Below is a list of the most effective plants and how to use them:

- **Aloe Vera**: Aloe vera is a plant widely celebrated for its soothing, anti-inflammatory, and healing properties, making it an excellent choice for alleviating the discomfort associated with hemorrhoids.

For external hemorrhoids, it is recommended to thoroughly cleanse the affected area and apply fresh aloe vera pulp directly onto the skin several times a day, preferably after bowel movements. Its cooling properties provide immediate relief from itching, burning, and inflammation.

For internal hemorrhoids, aloe vera gel is equally effective. To use it, extract the pure gel from the plant, place it inside a clean straw, and freeze it. Once frozen, cut a small piece and use it as a suppository, gently inserting it into the anus. This method, when performed once or twice daily, helps reduce inflammation and pain while promoting faster recovery.

‣ In addition to aloe vera, several other medicinal plants are highly effective in relieving hemorrhoid symptoms when used topically. Preparing these remedies is simple: create a concentrated infusion from the plant of your choice, allow it to cool completely, and soak a piece of gauze in the solution. Apply the gauze to the cleansed area for several minutes to achieve a soothing and restorative effect.

Likewise, these plants are also ideal for preparing sitz baths, which can be used to treat both external and internal hemorrhoids. Below are the main recommended plants and their properties:

‣ **Chamomile:** Known for its anti-inflammatory and soothing properties, chamomile helps relieve itching, burning, and inflammation. It is ideal for sensitive skin and can be used frequently without the risk of irritation.

‣ **Witch Hazel:** This powerful natural astringent reduces swelling, soothes pain, and promotes healing. Its cooling effect makes it an excellent option for external hemorrhoids.

‣ **Horse Chestnut:** Horse chestnut improves blood circulation and strengthens blood vessel walls, reducing inflammation and pain. It is particularly beneficial for hemorrhoids linked to circulatory issues.

‣ **Horsetail:** Thanks to its healing and vasoconstrictive properties, horsetail is very effective in stopping minor bleeding and accelerating recovery in the affected area.

Each of these plants can be used individually or combined to enhance their effects. Sitz baths, besides being a comfortable way to apply these therapeutic properties, relax the tissues and improve blood flow in the area, providing significant and lasting relief.

‣ **How to Take a Sitz Bath:** Start by preparing a concentrated infusion using one of the recommended plants. Once ready, let the infusion cool so that it is not hot when it comes into contact with the skin.

Add the infusion to a few inches of warm water in the bathtub, a large container, or a bidet.

Sit comfortably, immersing the affected area, and bend your knees toward your chest. This position promotes better blood circulation in the area, helping to reduce inflammation, relieve itching, and speed up the healing process for both external and internal hemorrhoids.

It is recommended to perform sitz baths for 15 to 20 minutes, 2 to 3 times a day, especially after bowel movements or whenever you experience significant discomfort.

This simple treatment will provide quick and natural relief, promoting the regeneration of the affected tissues.

Effective Plants for Internal Use

The most effective medicinal plants for treating hemorrhoids, presented in alphabetical order, are: **Aloe vera, horse chestnut, ginkgo biloba, witch hazel, chamomile, butcher's broom, and red vine.** Below, you will find a detailed description of each plant, including the various ways to consume them and the recommended dosages. Scientific names are provided in parentheses, as many of these plants may be known by different common names in various parts of the world.

Important: It is strongly recommended to consume infusions or decoctions in their natural form, without any sweeteners, in order to preserve their full medicinal properties. However, if you prefer to sweeten them, choose only 100% natural stevia as your option.

For optimal results, select one plant and consume it consistently for the recommended duration, or at least for a minimum of three weeks. If you do not observe significant improvement after this period, you may switch to another plant to find the one that best suits your needs. This approach allows you to take advantage of the unique therapeutic properties of each plant while adapting to your body's response.

Aloe Vera (Aloe barbadensis)

When consumed internally, aloe gel has anti-inflammatory and healing properties that help reduce inflammation and promote the healing of hemorrhoids.

Aloe vera gel with honey. Ingredients: 2 tablespoons of aloe vera gel and 1 tablespoon of honey. Preparation: Extract the gel from a ripe aloe vera leaf. Mix the aloe vera gel with the honey in a bowl. Stir well until a homogeneous mixture is obtained. Take a spoonful of this mixture after the main meals.

Butcher's Broom (Ruscus aculeatus)

Butcher's broom has venotonic and anti-inflammatory properties. It helps strengthen blood vessels and reduces inflammation.

Decoction (with the root): Ingredients: 35 grams of root per liter of water. Put the root in the water and boil for 10 minutes. Drink warm and unsweetened or with stevia. Consume 3 cups a day between meals.

Consume for a maximum of 8 weeks and then rest for 4 weeks.

Chamomile (Chamaemelum nobile)

It has anti-inflammatory and soothing properties. It helps to relieve pain and inflammation.

Infusion: Ingredients: 1 teaspoon of dried chamomile flowers and optionally honey. Boil 1 cup of water in a saucepan and then reduce the heat. Add the chamomile and simmer for 1 minute. Remove from heat and let steep for 2 more minutes. Pour the infusion into a cup, drink it alone, or add a little honey.

Ginger (Zingiber officinale)

Ginger is beneficial for hemorrhoids due to its anti-inflammatory properties, ability to improve circulation, analgesic action and digestive effect.

Infusion: Ingredients: fresh ginger root, about 2-3 centimeters, and 1 cup of water. First, peel and thinly slice the ginger root. Then, boil the water in a saucepan and add the slices. Let it cook for about 5 to 10 minutes over medium-low heat. Then, remove the saucepan from the heat and let the infusion steep to remove the pieces of ginger. You can add honey or lemon.

Ginkgo Biloba (Ginkgo biloba L.)

This plant has been used in traditional medicine to improve blood circulation and strengthen blood vessels.

Infusion: Ingredients: 50 grams of dried leaves in 500 ml of water. Boil the water, add the ginkgo, and let it steep for 8 minutes. Sweeten with honey or stevia. Drink 3 cups a day between meals.

Consume this infusion for a maximum of 8 weeks and then rest for 4 weeks.

Horse Chestnut (Aesculus hippocastanum)

This plant has been traditionally used to treat circulatory problems, including hemorrhoids. It improves blood circulation and strengthens blood vessels.

Decoction: The ingredients are 30 grams (2 tablespoons) of dried horse chestnut bark and 1 liter of water. To prepare it, heat the water and add the horse chestnut once the water is boiling. Let it cook for 10 minutes. Please remove it from the heat and let it cool. Consume it without sweeteners or sweeten it with pure stevia or honey. Please take it in two or three doses a day after meals.

Consume this decoction for a maximum of 4 weeks, then rest for 3 weeks. During this rest period, you can try another of the plants recommended in this book.

Red Vine (Vitis vinifera)

Red Vine is known for its vagotonic properties, strengthening blood vessels and improving circulation. Consuming it helps reduce inflammation and discomfort associated with hemorrhoids.

Decoction: The ingredients are 3 tablespoons of shredded dried leaves per liter of water. To prepare it, put the leaves in the water and heat them. Let it boil for 15 minutes. Drink 2 or 3 glasses a day between meals.

Decoction No. 2 (for acute hemorrhoid crisis): Ingredients: 1 teaspoon of dried leaves per cup of water. Preparation: Place the leaves in the water and boil for 10 minutes. Remove from the heat and let it stand for 10 more minutes. Take 1 tablespoon every 15 minutes. This recipe helps reduce the swelling of hemorrhoids.

Consume this decoction for up to 8 weeks and then rest for 4 weeks.

Witch Hazel (Hamamelis virginiana)

This plant has anti-inflammatory and astringent properties that help reduce the inflammation of hemorrhoids.

Infusion: Add 1 teaspoon of dried witch hazel to 1 cup of water. Heat the water until it boils. When it does, turn off the heat and add the witch hazel. Cover and let stand for 10 to 15 minutes–drink unsweetened or with stevia. Consume 2 cups a day between meals.

Consume for a maximum of 8 weeks and then rest for 4 weeks.

Herbal Remedy Recipes

While the plants mentioned above are effective when used individually, their properties can be significantly enhanced when combined correctly. Below are some particularly effective combinations:

▸ **Herbal Remedy Recipe No. 1**

The ingredients are witch hazel, ginkgo biloba, horse chestnut, and butcher's broom. Use the four plants in equal parts.

Preparation: Add 2 teaspoons of this mixture of dried herbs to 500 ml of water. Heat the water with the plants and let it come to a boil for 3 minutes. Remove it from the heat and allow it to steep for 15 minutes. Drink this infusion throughout the day.

▸ **Herbal Remedy Recipe No. 2**

The ingredients are red vine leaves, chamomile flowers, and mullein leaves. Use the three plants in equal parts.

Preparation: Boil 1 cup of water. Add the witch hazel leaves, horsetail, and chamomile to the hot water. Let the infusion steep for 10-15 minutes. Strain the liquid. If desired, sweeten with honey.

Simple Steps to Make a Tincture for Hemorrhoids

Tinctures, also known as concentrated botanical extracts, are an effective and potent way to harness the therapeutic benefits of medicinal plants. Through a careful extraction process, essential compounds, such as phytochemicals and active principles, are obtained, providing valuable healing properties.

These liquid solutions have been used for centuries in traditional medicine due to their proven efficacy and exceptional versatility. In recent years, they have regained their relevance thanks to the growing interest in natural remedies and herbal practices.

The method for preparing these extracts can vary, but it generally involves immersing plant parts–such as roots, leaves, flowers, or bark–in a solvent like alcohol, glycerin, or water. During the steeping process, the plant's active elements are extracted into the liquid, creating a medicinal concentrate that retains its essential properties.

One of the main advantages of these preparations is their practicality. They can be administered orally by adding a few drops to water or juice, allowing for rapid absorption. Additionally, their high concentration enables precise dosage adjustments based on individual needs.

> **Making a Butcher's Broom Tincture:**

Ingredients:
- 40 grams of butcher's broom root.
- 200 ml vodka or brandy (apple cider vinegar or vegetable glycerin can be used instead for those who cannot consume alcohol)
- A glass bottle of approximately 200 ml with an airtight cap
- A bottle with a dark brown dropper to protect it from the light

Preparation:
1. Peel the butternut squash and slice or grate it. Place the broom in an airtight glass jar, filling about half of the jar.
2. Fill the jar with vodka, brandy, or vinegar. Shake well to ensure a good mixture.
3. Store the jar in a dark, warm place away from heat sources. Let the mixture macerate for at least 3 weeks, although it can also be left to macerate for several months. Be sure to shake the jar once a week and put it away again.
4. After the maceration time, filter the tincture using sterilized cotton gauze in a glass container.
5. Transfer the filtered tincture to the brown glass dropper bottle and seal tightly. Label the bottle with the bottling date.

Dosage: The recommended dose for adults is 30 drops, 3 times daily, for a maximum of 4 consecutive weeks. After this period, a one-month break (4 weeks of treatment and 1 month break) is recommended before continuing.

Storage: Keep the tincture in a cool, dark place, and make sure to check the expiration date (1 year).

Learn Everything You Need to Know About the Plants

In this section, we'll delve into the most recommended

botanical species for treating the condition at hand. You'll find essential information about their possible adverse effects, contraindications, and interactions, as well as detailed insights into each plant. From their descriptions and habitats to their uses, chemical components, histories, and therapeutic properties, this chapter is designed to take you on a fascinating journey of discovery.

My goal is to provide you with a comprehensive understanding of these plants, helping you grasp their context and fully appreciate their many benefits. We'll explore their historical origins and significance in traditional medicine, highlighting their invaluable role in natural care.

I want you to become an expert on these species, capable of making informed decisions in your pursuit of wellness. Get ready to expand your knowledge and uncover the extraordinary healing power of nature!

Aloe Vera (Aloe barbadensis)

Description:
Aloe vera, also known as aloe vera, is a perennial succulent plant in the lily family. Its leaves are fleshy and lanceolate, growing in a rosette.

Habitat and cultivation:
Aloe vera thrives in warm, dry climates, preferably with temperatures between 20 and 30 degrees Celsius. It requires well-drained soils and does not tolerate excess moisture. It reproduces using leaf cuttings and can be grown in pots or gardens.

Parts used:
The main parts used by Aloe vera are the leaves. These contain a transparent gel obtained by cutting and opening the fresh leaves. The dried leaves and the yellow sap under the leaves' skin are also occasionally used.

Components:
Aloe gel contains polysaccharides, vitamins (such as C and E), minerals (such as magnesium, calcium, and zinc), enzymes, amino acids, and antioxidants, contributing to its therapeutic properties.

History and tradition:
Aloe vera has a rich history of use. It was known in ancient Egypt as "the plant of immortality" and has been used in traditional Chinese and Ayurvedic medicine. Over the centuries, its reputation as a medicinal plant has gained worldwide recognition.

Therapeutic properties:
Aloe vera treats burns, wounds, insect bites, and skin conditions such as psoriasis and acne. It has also been used to relieve skin irritation and inflammation. Consumption of Aloe vera juice is associated with digestive health benefits, relieving constipation and promoting intestinal health.

Curiosities:
Aloe vera has some interesting curiosities associated with its history and use. For example, it is believed that Cleopatra used Aloe vera gel as part of her beauty routine. In World War II, aloe gel was used as a blood substitute in emergencies, as its chemical composition resembled that of blood plasma. It has also been used in the food industry as an additive in yogurts and beverages.

Adverse or side effects:
Although Aloe vera is generally safe for topical use and moderate oral consumption, some people may experience adverse effects. Some people may have allergic reactions or skin irritation when applying Aloe vera gel. In rare cases, excessive consumption of Aloe juice may cause abdominal cramps, diarrhea and electrolyte imbalances. In addition, it has been reported that prolonged use of high concentrations of Aloe vera on the skin may cause dryness and flaking.

Contraindications:
Although Aloe vera is considered safe for most people, some contraindications exist. It is not recommended for topical use on deep wounds, severe burns, or open surgical wounds, as it may delay healing. In addition, pregnant and nursing women should consult a healthcare professional before using Aloe vera products, as there may be potential risks to the fetus or baby.

Interactions:
Aloe vera may interact with certain medications and supplements, so it is essential to exercise caution when using it in combination with other products. For example, consuming Aloe vera may increase the risk of bleeding in people taking anticoagulants such as warfarin. It has also been reported that Aloe vera may interfere with the absorption of oral medications,

such as angiotensin-converting enzyme inhibitors (ACE inhibitors) used to treat high blood pressure.

Butcher's Broom (Ruscus aculeatus)

Description:
Butcher's broom is a perennial plant in the Liliaceae family. It is native to Europe and parts of Asia and is characterized as a shrub with stiff, evergreen leaves. Its stems are green and branched, and the leaves have needle-like thorns, which have earned it the common name of spicy butcher's broom. The plant produces small greenish flowers and red berries.

Habitat and cultivation:
Butcher's broom grows best in wooded and shady areas with moist, well-drained soils. It is commonly found in oak, beech, and pine forests. However, it can also be grown in gardens and containers. It prefers acidic soils and partial or complete shade.

Parts used:
The roots and rhizomes are mainly used medicinally. These parts of the plant contain various beneficial compounds that provide therapeutic properties.

Components:
Butcher's broom contains several active components, including steroids, saponins, flavonoids and tannins. These compounds are responsible for the plant's medicinal properties.

History and tradition:
Traditional European medicine has long used it. Since ancient times, it has been valued for its diuretic, anti-inflammatory, and vagotonic properties. In addition, it has been used to treat circulatory problems, such as venous insufficiency and hemorrhoids.

Therapeutic properties:
It is used in phytotherapy due to its therapeutic properties. It is attributed to benefits such as improving blood circulation, strengthening veins and capillaries, reducing inflammation, and relieving symptoms of hemorrhoids. It has also been used to treat lymphatic system disorders and relieve symptoms of tired legs and varicose veins.

Curiosities:

Butcher's broom is associated with some exciting curiosities. For example, although it is called hot because of the thorns on its leaves, it does not belong to the family of hot plants like chili peppers. Also, the red berries of butcher's broom are poisonous to humans, so they should not be consumed.

Adverse or side effects:
Although butcher's broom is generally safe when used properly, some mild adverse effects have been reported in isolated cases. These may include stomach upset, nausea, diarrhea, or allergic reactions in sensitive people. If any side effects are experienced, use should be discontinued.

Contraindications:
Although it is considered safe for most people, some contraindications should be considered. Its use is not recommended in pregnant or breastfeeding women due to the lack of sufficient evidence on its safety in these stages. In addition, people with kidney or heart disorders, as well as those taking anticoagulant medications, should avoid using butcher's brooms without consulting a physician.

Interactions:
It may interact with certain medications and herbs, so caution is essential when combining it with other treatments. It may potentiate the effects of anticoagulant drugs, such as warfarin, increasing the risk of bleeding. In addition, it may interfere with iron absorption, so it is recommended to separate the intake of iron supplements from the intake of butcher's broom.

Calendula (Calendula officinalis)

Description:
Calendula, scientifically known as Calendula officinalis, is an annual or biennial herbaceous plant belonging to the Asteraceae family. It is characterized by light green, lanceolate leaves and large, showy flowers, usually bright yellow or orange. Marigold flowers are similar in appearance to daisies, with reed-shaped petals and a center filled with small tubular flowers.

Habitat and cultivation:
Calendula is native to the Mediterranean region but has naturalized in many parts of the world. It prefers to grow in temperate, sunny climates, although it can tolerate partial shade. It adapts well to different types of well-drained soils and is

commonly found in gardens, fields and meadows.

As for cultivation, marigolds can be grown from seeds sown in spring or autumn. Direct sowing in the ground or pots is recommended at a depth of about 1 cm. The plant is hardy and easy to care for, requiring regular but moderate watering. It flowers during summer and autumn, and its flowers can be harvested for use.

Parts used:
The parts of the marigold used are mainly the flowers. These are harvested when they are fully open and in full bloom. The flowers are dried and used in various forms, such as infusions, oils, ointments, or tinctures. They can also be used fresh in salads or other dishes.

Components:
It contains various beneficial components, including flavonoids, carotenoids, essential oils, phenolic acids, and triterpenes, which give the plant its medicinal and antioxidant properties.

History and tradition:
Calendula has a long history of use in folk medicine and herbal traditions. It has been prized for its medicinal properties and used to treat many conditions, including wounds, burns, skin inflammations, digestive problems and gynecological ailments. In addition, calendula has been considered a symbol of joy and prosperity in many cultures and is used in celebrations and rituals.

Therapeutic properties:
It is known for its therapeutic properties and health benefits. Some of the properties attributed to this plant include anti-inflammatory, healing, antiseptic, antioxidant, and soothing actions. It has been used topically to treat minor burns, cuts, abrasions, insect bites, eczema and dermatitis. Due to its moisturizing properties and ability to improve skin appearance, it has also been used in skin care products such as creams, lotions, and ointments.

Curiosities:
Calendula, also known as "marigold", is a medicinal plant widely used for its healing and cosmetic properties.

It is native to southern Europe, although it is currently cultivated in various regions of the world.

Its bright orange flowers are used both fresh and dried to prepare infusions, oils and creams.

Calendula has been used since ancient times for its anti-inflammatory, healing, and antioxidant properties.

It is commonly used in cosmetics to manufacture creams, lotions and skin care products.

Calendula is used externally and as an infusion to treat digestive problems and regulate the menstrual cycle.

In traditional medicine, it is attributed to antispasmodic, diuretic, and emmenagogue properties.

Adverse or side effects:
In general, calendula is considered safe for topical use or as an infusion. However, there are some possible adverse effects:

Some people may experience allergic reactions such as redness, irritation, or skin itching.

In rare cases, severe allergic reactions, such as swelling of the face, lips, or tongue, difficulty breathing, or extensive skin rashes, have been reported. If these symptoms occur, medical attention should be sought immediately.

Contraindications:
Although calendula is considered safe for most people, there are some contraindications to be aware of.

People allergic to plants in the Asteraceae family, such as chrysanthemum, arnica, or daisy, may be more likely to develop allergic reactions to calendula and should avoid using it.

In case of pregnancy or breastfeeding, it is recommended to consult a health professional before using calendula products, as there is not enough evidence of its safety in these stages.

If surgery is scheduled, calendula should be avoided, as it may interfere with blood clotting.

Interactions:
No significant interactions between calendula and specific medications have been reported. However, it is always advisable to consult a physician or pharmacist before combining calendula with other medicines, such as:

Caution is crucial if you are taking anticoagulant drugs, such as warfarin, as this may increase the risk of bleeding.

Caution is also advised if you are taking medication for diabetes, as calendula may lower blood sugar levels.

Chamomile (Matricaria chamomilla)

Description:
Chamomile is an annual herbaceous plant in the Asteraceae family. Its erect, branched stem can reach a height of up to 60 centimeters. The leaves are finely divided and light green. The flowers are small and daisy-shaped, with a yellow center surrounded by white petals. A distinctive apple scent is released when the flowers are rubbed between the fingers.

Habitat and cultivation:
Chamomile is native to Europe and commonly found in temperate climate regions. It grows best in well-drained, nutrient-rich soils and can be found in meadows, fields, roadsides and gardens. Chamomile is a hardy and adaptable plant that can grow in various conditions. It can also be quickly grown from seed or by dividing existing plants.

Parts used:
The dried flowers are used in the chamomile parts. These are harvested when fully open and air-dried to preserve their therapeutic properties. The dried flowers are used to prepare infusions, extracts, essential oils and cosmetic products.

Components:
Chamomile contains various components that contribute to its therapeutic properties. These include essential oils, such as bisabolol and azulene oxide, which have anti-inflammatory and soothing properties. It also contains flavonoids, such as apigenin, which have antioxidant and anti-inflammatory properties. Other components present in chamomile include caffeic acid, coumarins and polyphenols.

History and tradition:
Various cultures have utilized chamomile since ancient times due to its therapeutic properties. The ancient Egyptians employed it in religious rituals and skincare applications. It was also recognized and utilized in traditional Greek and Roman medicine. In popular tradition, chamomile is associated with

calming and relaxing properties, and it has been used to relieve stress, anxiety, and sleep disorders.

Therapeutic properties:
Chamomile is known for its therapeutic properties and is used in herbal medicine for its various health benefits. It has anti-inflammatory, antioxidant, antibacterial, soothing, and digestive properties. Chamomile is commonly used to relieve upset stomach, colic, indigestion and nausea. It is also used to reduce stress and anxiety and promote relaxation. In addition, it has been used topically to relieve skin irritation, minor burns, and skin conditions such as dermatitis and eczema.

Curiosities:
Chamomile (Matricaria chamomilla) is an herbaceous Asteraceae plant with exciting curiosities. For example, its name comes from the Greek "chamaimelon", which means "apple on earth", due to its characteristic apple aroma. In addition, chamomile has been used for centuries in multiple cultures for its therapeutic properties and is considered one of the oldest and most popular herbs in herbal medicine.

Adverse or side effects:
Chamomile is generally considered safe and well-tolerated. However, adverse effects or side effects may occur in some cases. Some people may experience allergic reactions when they come into contact with the plant or consume chamomile products. In addition, excessive consumption of chamomile may cause stomach upset, nausea, or vomiting in some people. It is essential to be aware of these possible effects, discontinue use, and consult a health professional if you experience any.

Contraindications:
Although generally safe, it has some contraindications. For example, people who are allergic to other plants in the Asteraceae family, such as ragweed or sunflower, may be at increased risk of developing allergic reactions to chamomile. In addition, caution is advised in pregnant or nursing women, as not enough studies have been conducted to determine its safety during pregnancy and lactation.

Interactions:
In general, chamomile has not been associated with significant drug interactions. However, it is always advisable to consult a healthcare professional if you are taking any medications or have pre-existing health conditions before using chamomile thera-peutically. Some studies suggest that chamomile may have mild

anticoagulant effects, so caution should be exercised when combining it with anticoagulant or antiplatelet medications.

Ginger (Zingiber officinale)

Description:
Ginger is a perennial plant with underground stems called rhizomes. It has long, narrow leaves and yellow or white cone-shaped flowers. The rhizome is the most commonly used part and has a spicy and aromatic flavor.

Habitat and cultivation:
Ginger is native to tropical Asia and is grown in many parts of the world. It prefers warm, humid climates and can be grown both in gardens and in pots indoors.

Parts used:
The rhizome of ginger is the most commonly used part. It is harvested, peeled, and used fresh or dried for culinary and medicinal purposes. The leaves and flowers can also be used in specific preparations.

Components:
Ginger contains active compounds such as gingerol, shogaol and zingiberene, which give it medicinal properties. It also contains antioxidants, vitamins and minerals.

Ginger, scientifically known as Zingiber officinale, is a perennial plant native to tropical Asia. Due to its multiple health benefits, it has been used for centuries as a spice in cooking and traditional medicine.

History and tradition:
This plant has been cultivated and used in Asia for over 5,000 years. It is believed to have originated in the coastal regions of South Asia, specifically in what is today known as India and China. From there, it spread to various parts of the world and was integrated into the culinary and medicinal traditions of many cultures.

Ginger is especially valued in traditional Asian medicine, such as Ayurvedic and Chinese medicine. In these traditions, it is considered a "hot" plant that can help balance the body and treat various ailments. It has been used to relieve digestive problems, such as nausea, vomiting and upset stomach. In addition, it has been used as a general tonic to strengthen the immune system and promote blood circulation.

Therapeutic properties:
Ginger contains bioactive compounds, such as gingerols and shogaols, which give it medicinal properties. These compounds are responsible for ginger's characteristic flavor and aroma and have health benefits for the human body.

One of ginger's best-known properties is its ability to relieve nausea and vomiting. Numerous studies have shown that ginger consumption can effectively relieve nausea caused by pregnancy, chemotherapy, or surgery. The compounds in ginger act on the digestive system, reducing discomfort and improving intestinal motility.

In addition, ginger has also been used to relieve pain and inflammation. Gingerols and shogaols have been shown to have anti-inflammatory and analgesic properties, making them a natural choice for pain relief in conditions such as arthritis, muscle aches and migraines. Some studies even suggest that regular consumption of ginger may help reduce chronic inflammation in the body.

Ginger also has positive effects on cardiovascular health. Regular consumption can help reduce cholesterol and triglyceride levels in the blood and improve blood circulation, which could contribute to heart health and reduce the risk of cardiovascular disease.

In addition to its therapeutic properties, ginger is also used as a spice in cooking due to its spicy and aromatic flavor. It is added to savory and sweet dishes, as well as to beverages such as ginger tea. Its culinary versatility makes it popular in many cultures and cuisines worldwide.

Curiosities:
Ginger is a plant native to tropical Asia. It has been used for centuries in cooking and traditional medicine due to its medicinal properties. Here are some interesting facts about ginger:

Spicy and refreshing flavor: Ginger has a distinctive taste and a refreshing touch. This characteristic flavor is due to active compounds such as gingerols and shogaols, which also give it its medicinal properties.

Ancient use: Ginger has been used in traditional Chinese and Indian medicine for over 2,000 years to treat various conditions, from digestive problems to muscle aches and colds.

Culinary use: Ginger is a trendy cooking spice. Besides its medicinal properties, it is used in sweet and savory dishes, such as curries, desserts, infusions, and refreshing drinks like ginger ale.

Adverse or side effects:
Although ginger is generally safe for most people when consumed in moderate amounts, some people may experience adverse side effects:

Upset stomach: Excessive consumption of ginger may cause an upset stomach, nausea, heartburn, or diarrhea in some people. These side effects are usually mild and go away on their own.

Interference with medications: Ginger may interact with certain drugs, such as anticoagulants or antihypertensives. When combining ginger with these drugs, caution is advised; it is crucial to consult a physician.

Allergic reactions: Although rare, some people may be allergic to ginger. These reactions may manifest as skin rashes, itching, swelling, or difficulty breathing. If you experience any allergic reactions, seek medical attention immediately.

Contraindications:
There are contraindications to take into account when using ginger:

Coagulation disorders: Because ginger inhibits platelet aggregation, caution should be exercised in people with coagulation disorders or who take anticoagulant drugs. A physician should be consulted before use.

Pregnancy and lactation: Although ginger has traditionally been used to treat morning sickness, it should be used cautiously during pregnancy and lactation. A physician should be consulted before using it during these stages.

Interactions:
Ginger can interact with certain medications and supplements, so it is essential to use caution when combining it with other treatments. Some known interactions include:

Anticoagulants: Ginger, which inhibits platelet aggregation, may increase the risk of bleeding when combined with anticoagulant medications such as warfarin. Medical supervision is recommended if both treatments are used.

Antihypertensives: Ginger may have hypotensive effects, which could interact with high blood pressure medications. If you are taking medicines for hypertension, exercise caution and consult a physician before using ginger.

Ginkgo (Ginkgo biloba)

Description:
Ginkgo biloba is an ancient tree that has existed for millions of years. It is considered a living fossil because of its unique appearance, which includes fan-shaped leaves and spreading branches. The tree can reach a height of up to 30 meters and has smooth, grayish bark. Its leaves are bright green in summer and turn golden in autumn before falling.

Habitat and cultivation:
Ginkgo biloba originated in China and has been cultivated in Asia for centuries. Today, it is found in many parts of the world, including Europe and North America. It prefers temperate climates and adapts well to different soil types. It is a hardy tree that can grow in urban and rural areas.

Parts used:
In medicinal terms, Ginkgo biloba's main parts are its leaves and seeds. The leaves are harvested in autumn and dried for later use. The seeds, on the other hand, are used to a lesser extent and must be processed appropriately, as they contain toxic substances when raw.

Components:
Ginkgo biloba contains a variety of active constituents, the most notable being flavonoids and terpenoids. Flavonoids are known for their antioxidant properties, while terpenoids, such as ginkgolides and bilobalides, have neuroprotective effects and improve blood circulation.

History and tradition:
Ginkgo biloba has a rich history and a long tradition in Chinese medicine. It has been used for centuries to treat memory, respiratory, and circulatory disorders. In addition, the Ginkgo

tree is considered sacred in some cultures, and spiritual and longevity properties are attributed to it.

Therapeutic properties:
Ginkgo biloba has been widely studied for its therapeutic properties. It improves blood circulation and oxygen flow to the brain, which may benefit memory and cognitive function. It has also been used to treat vision problems, tinnitus (ringing in the ears), and vertigo. However, it is essential to note that Ginkgo biloba supplements have side effects and may interact with certain medications.

Curiosities:
Ginkgo biloba is a fascinating species with several curiosities associated with it. For example, it is considered a "living fossil" because it has survived for millions of years without significant changes in its structure. In addition, it is a highly resistant tree, capable of surviving pollution, diseases and adverse weather conditions. It is also interesting to note that Ginkgo biloba leaves have a unique shape and are used in Chinese culture to prepare traditional dishes.

Adverse or side effects:
Although Ginkgo biloba is generally safe for most people when consumed adequately, some adverse effects may occur in rare cases. These side effects may include headaches, stomach upset, dizziness, diarrhea, nausea, or allergic reactions in some people. In addition, due to its anticoagulant effect, there is a risk of excessive bleeding in people who are taking anticoagulants or have clotting disorders. Caution is advised in people with seizures, clotting disorders, or those undergoing surgery.

Contraindications:
Although Ginkgo biloba is widely used, some contraindications should be considered. It is not recommended for pregnant or lactating women due to the lack of evidence on its safety in these cases. People with a known allergy to Ginkgo biloba or its components should also avoid it. Caution should also be exercised in people with seizure disorders, coagulation disorders, or who are scheduled for surgery soon, as Ginkgo may interact with drugs and increase the risk of complications.

Interactions:
Ginkgo may interact with certain medications, which may affect their effectiveness or increase the risk of adverse effects. For example, it may increase the risk of bleeding when taken with anticoagulants such as warfarin or aspirin. In addition, it

may interfere with the action of certain drugs used to treat seizure disorders, such as carbamazepine. It may also interact with drugs that affect liver function, such as some antidepressants and HIV medications. Therefore, informing your doctor or pharmacist if you are taking Ginkgo biloba is vital to avoid possible harmful interactions.

Horse Chestnut (Aesculus hippocastanum)

Description:
The horse chestnut is a medium-to-large tree that can reach a height of up to 30 meters. It has a straight trunk and spreading branches that form a rounded crown. Its leaves are large, compound, and palmate in shape, with 5 to 7 leaflets and serrated edges. During the spring, the tree produces flowers in the form of erect white or pale pink spikes. The fruits of the horse chestnut are spiny capsules containing shiny, dark brown seeds.

Habitat and cultivation:
Horse chestnut is native to the Balkans and Asia Minor mountain regions but is now cultivated in many parts of the world. It prefers temperate to cool climates and well-drained soils. Horse chestnuts are commonly found in parks, avenues, and gardens, and their wood is also used for furniture and flooring.

Parts used:
Regarding therapeutic use, the most used parts of horse chestnut are the seeds and the bark. The most valued seeds are used to prepare extracts and tinctures. The bark can also be used as a decoction or tincture.

Components:
Horse chestnut seeds contain various compounds, among which triterpene saponosides, such as escin, stand out. Escin is considered the main active component responsible for the therapeutic properties of horse chestnut. Flavonoids, tannins and other bioactive compounds are also found in smaller quantities.

History and tradition:
Horse chestnut has been used in herbal medicine for centuries. It is believed to have been introduced to Europe from Asia in the 16th century. Traditionally, it has been used to treat circulatory problems such as venous insufficiency, varicose veins and

capillary fragility. It has also been used topically to relieve inflammation and pain related to bruises, contusions and hematomas.

Therapeutic properties:
Horse chestnut is mainly used for its vagotonic and vasoprotective properties. The escin in the seeds can strengthen blood vessels, improve circulation, and reduce inflammation. Thus, it is a popular natural remedy for treating venous disorders such as varicose veins, chronic venous insufficiency and heavy legs.

In addition to its venotonic properties, horse chestnut has antioxidant and anti-inflammatory effects.

Curiosities:
Horse chestnut is scientifically known as Aesculus hippocastanum. The Latin word "Aesculus" refers to a type of oak tree, while "hippocastanum" means "horse chestnut". The latter name is derived from the ancient tradition of feeding the tree's seeds to horses.

Although it is known as "horse chestnut", this plant has no relation to the common chestnut. Its name is derived from the fact that the Portuguese colonizers brought it to Europe from Asia, and it was mistakenly associated with the East Indies.

In some cultures, especially in Eastern Europe, horse chestnut seeds have historically been used to make amulets and talismans that were believed to protect against the evil eye and other negative energies.

Adverse or side effects:
Although horse chestnut is generally well tolerated, adverse effects may occur.

Some people may experience stomach upset, nausea, vomiting, and headache. These side effects are usually mild and go away on their own.

In rare cases, allergic reactions have been reported. If you experience symptoms such as rash, itching, swelling, or difficulty breathing after consumption, it is vital to seek medical attention immediately.

Contraindications:
People with liver or kidney disease, as well as those with bleeding disorders or gastric ulcers, should avoid the use of horse

chestnut, as it may worsen these conditions.

Due to its ability to affect blood coagulation, horse chestnut should be used cautiously in people who are taking anticoagulants or antiplatelet drugs, such as warfarin. In these cases, it is essential to consult a physician before use.

Interactions:
Horse chestnuts may interact with certain medications, such as anticoagulants, antiplatelets, and nonsteroidal anti-inflammatory drugs (NSAIDs). It may increase the risk of bleeding or interfere with the effectiveness of these medications. If you take any of them, you must talk to your doctor before taking horse chestnut.

In addition, it has been reported that it may interact with blood pressure medications, diuretics, and medications that affect liver function. Therefore, it is advisable to consult a health professional before combining them.

Horsetail (Equisetum arvense)

Description:
Horsetail is a perennial plant belonging to the genus Equisetum. It is characterized by hollow, jointed stems that resemble horse tails. It has small leaves and cone-shaped spores at the top of the stems.

Habitat and cultivation:
Horsetail is commonly found in wet and marshy areas around the world. It grows in mineral-rich soils and can tolerate different light and water conditions. It can be grown in gardens and is also found in the wild.

Parts used:
The parts of horsetail used are the sterile stems that grow in spring before the appearance of spores. These stems are harvested and used fresh and dried to obtain their medicinal properties.

Components:
Horsetail contains several beneficial components, including silica, flavonoids, minerals (such as potassium and calcium), ascorbic acid (vitamin C), and alkaloids. Silica is a central component contributing to the plant's healing properties.

History and tradition:
Horsetail has been used in traditional medicine for centuries due to its medicinal properties and health benefits. It is a perennial plant in various parts of the world, including Europe, Asia and North America. Its name comes from its appearance, as its stems resemble horsetails.

This plant has been highly valued in the history and traditions of various cultures. In ancient Rome, for example, it was believed to possess healing properties and was used to treat wounds and urinary problems. Additionally, it was utilized in traditional Chinese and Indian Ayurvedic medicine to treat a range of ailments.

In addition to its medicinal uses, horsetail has also been used in agriculture and gardening due to its silica content. This substance strengthens plant tissues and promotes plant growth. Horsetail has also strengthened fabric fibers in cosmetic products and the textile industry.

Therapeutic properties:
Horsetail is known for its therapeutic properties and health benefits. Some of its most outstanding properties are:

Natural Diuretic: Horsetail has a mild diuretic effect, stimulating urine production and helping eliminate toxins and wastes from the body. This can be beneficial in treating fluid retention, reducing swelling, and promoting kidney health.

Strengthening bones and tissues: Horsetail contains silica, a mineral in high concentrations in this plant. Silica is essential for forming and strengthening connective tissues, such as bones, cartilage and nails. It can also help promote healthy skin, hair and teeth.

Anti-inflammatory properties: Its anti-inflammatory properties can help reduce inflammation in the body, which can be beneficial in treating inflammatory conditions such as arthritis and inflammatory bowel disease.

Improving urinary system health: Horsetail has traditionally been used to treat urinary tract infections and kidney stones. Its diuretic effect helps cleanse and detoxify the kidneys, promoting kidney health and preventing stone formation.

Antioxidant action: Horsetail contains antioxidants that help protect cells from damage caused by free radicals. Free radicals are unstable molecules that can damage DNA and contribute to aging and various diseases. The antioxidants in horsetail help neutralize these free radicals and protect the body against oxidative stress.

Curiosities:
Horsetail is a perennial herb that grows in wet, marshy areas worldwide. It gets its name because of its distinctive appearance, resembling a horsetail's bristles. In addition to its peculiar appearance, this plant has several interesting curiosities:

Living fossils: Horsetails are considered living fossils, as they are plants that have existed on Earth for millions of years. The first horsetail species is believed to have emerged more than 300 million years ago, during the Carboniferous period.

Silica content: It is one of the few plants that contains high levels of silica, an essential mineral for human health. This makes it a popular plant in traditional medicine for strengthening hair, nails and bones.

Use in gardening: Besides its medicinal properties, it is appreciated for its unique structure. Its hollow, jointed stems make it an ornamental plant in water gardens or for creating natural borders in flower beds.

Adverse or side effects:
Despite its potential benefits, horsetail may have some adverse effects in some instances, such as the following:

Thiaminase toxicity: Horsetail contains an enzyme called thiaminase, which can interfere with the absorption of vitamin B1 (thiamine). If consumed in large amounts or for prolonged periods, this can lead to thiamine deficiency in the body.

Interference with medications: Horsetail may interact with certain medications, such as diuretics or blood thinners. If you take any medication, consult a physician before using the plant to avoid negative interactions.

Allergic reactions: Some people may be allergic to horsetail. These reactions may manifest as rashes, itching, swelling, or difficulty breathing. If any allergic reaction occurs, immediate medical attention should be sought.

Contraindications:
There are contraindications to take into account when using

horsetail:

Pregnancy and lactation: The safety of horsetail during pregnancy and lactation has not been sufficiently investigated. As a precaution, pregnant or nursing women should avoid using it or consult a physician before using it.

Kidney problems: Due to its silica content and diuretic capacity, horsetail should be avoided by people with kidney problems, such as kidney stones or kidney failure, as it may aggravate these problems.

Interactions:
It can interact with certain medications and supplements, so it is essential to use caution when combining it with other treatments. Some known interactions include:

Diuretic medications: Horsetail has natural diuretic properties to increase the diuretic effect of diuretic medicines. This could lead to excessive fluid and mineral loss in the body.

Anticoagulants: They may have mild anticoagulant effects, which could increase the risk of bleeding when combined with anticoagulant drugs such as warfarin. Medical supervision is recommended if both treatments are used.

Red Vine (Vitis vinifera)

The red vine is a climbing plant in the Vitaceae family. It is known for its deep red grapes and use in wine production.

Description:
The red vine is a perennial plant that can grow to considerable heights, reaching over 10 meters in length under favorable conditions. Its leaves are large, lobed, and have serrated edges. During autumn, the leaves take on reddish tones, which gives them their common name. The bunches of grapes the red vine produces are small and contain round or ellipsoidal dark red or purple berries.

Habitat and cultivation:
The red vine is native to the Mediterranean region but is now cultivated in many parts of the world. It requires a temperate climate and well-drained soils to grow appropriately. The vine is mainly grown for its grapes, which are used in wine production

and can also be consumed fresh.

Parts used:
The leaves and grapes are the most commonly used parts of the red vine for therapeutic purposes. The leaves are harvested during the summer and dried for later use in infusions and extracts, while the grapes can also be used to prepare home remedies.

Components:
Red vine leaves contain several bioactive compounds, including flavonoids like quercetin and rutin. These compounds are known for their antioxidant and anti-inflammatory properties. Tannins, organic acids, and minerals such as potassium and calcium are also found in the leaves.

History and tradition:
Humans have cultivated and used the red vine for thousands of years. Its cultivation dates back to ancient Mesopotamia and Egypt, where it was prized for its grapes and symbolic and ceremonial value. Throughout history, the red vine has been associated with celebration, good health and longevity.

Therapeutic properties:
Due to its therapeutic properties, it has traditionally been used in herbal medicine. It helps improve blood circulation, strengthen capillary vessels, and reduce capillary fragility and permeability. It is also attributed with antioxidant and anti-inflammatory properties, which may contribute to cardiovascular health and alleviate symptoms of circulatory disorders such as varicose veins and venous insufficiency.

Curiosities:
The red vine is one of the oldest plants humans have cultivated. Its cultivation dates back more than 6,000 years.

Red vine grapes are used in wine production, herbal medicine, juices, jams and other gastronomic products.

The red vine is a vigorous climbing plant and can cover large areas, forming dense vines in vineyards.

Adverse or side effects:
Although red vine is generally considered safe, mild adverse effects, such as stomach upset, nausea, or diarrhea, may sometimes occur. These side effects are uncommon and are usually temporary.

Some people may have allergic reactions to red vine. If you experience itching, swelling, or difficulty breathing after consumption, seek medical attention immediately.

Contraindications:
Red Vines have anticoagulant and antiplatelet effects, which can interfere with blood clotting. Therefore, people taking anticoagulant or antiplatelet drugs, such as warfarin, should avoid excessive consumption of red vines or consult their physician before doing so.

Due to insufficient information, red vines should be used cautiously during pregnancy and lactation. Before using them during these stages, consult a health professional.

Interactions:
Red vine may interact with certain medications, such as anticoagulants, antiplatelets, nonsteroidal anti-inflammatory drugs (NSAIDs), and blood pressure medications. It may potentiate the effects of these medications, which may increase the risk of bleeding or affect the effectiveness of blood pressure medications. If you take any of these medications, you must talk to your doctor before consuming red vine.

Witch Hazel (Hamamelis virginiana)

Description:
Witch hazel is a shrub or small tree native to North America. It is characterized by its showy flowers and colorful foliage in autumn. Witch hazel has alternate, simple, toothed leaves, and its flowers are bright yellow or orange. It is known for its ability to bloom in winter and early spring, making it a popular ornamental plant.

Habitat and cultivation:
Witch hazel is found naturally in moist forests and swamps of North America, mainly in the eastern and central regions of the United States. It prefers humus-rich, well-drained soils. As for cultivation, it can be planted in gardens and parks, as long as it is provided with a suitable environment with partial shade and moist soil. It is a hardy plant and can tolerate cold temperatures.

Parts used:
In medicinal terms, Witch hazel is mainly used for its leaves and bark. The leaves are harvested in autumn and dried for later

use. The bark is obtained from young branches and dried for use. These parts contain active compounds with therapeutic properties.

Components:
Witch hazel contains various beneficial components, including tannins, flavonoids and volatile oils. Tannins are astringent and help reduce inflammation and skin irritation. Flavonoids possess antioxidant and anti-inflammatory properties, and volatile oils give the plant a distinctive aroma.

History and tradition:
Witch Hazel has a long history of use in traditional medicine. Native Americans, such as the Iroquois and Mohicans, used it to treat various conditions, including skin problems, hemorrhoids and muscle pain. It was also used in rituals and ceremonies. Today, witch hazel has become popular in skin care products and is used in topical treatments to soothe irritation and promote healing.

Therapeutic properties:
Witch hazel has long been used for its therapeutic properties, which include astringent, anti-inflammatory, and hemostatic action. It is commonly used to relieve discomforts such as insect bites, sunburn, rashes and irritated skin. Due to its ability to reduce inflammation and ease discomfort, witch hazel is also used to treat hemorrhoids. In addition, it can help stimulate blood circulation and promote the healing of minor wounds.

Curiosities:
It is a plant with some interesting curiosities associated with it. For example, it is known as the "witches' tree" because of its ability to bloom in the dead of winter, considered a magical power in ancient times. In addition, its flowers are unique, with slender, ribbon-like petals that curve back, giving them a distinctive appearance. It is also interesting to note that witch hazel is used in the cosmetic industry and is found in various skin care products due to its beneficial properties.

Adverse or side effects:
Although it is generally safe for most people when used topically, some adverse effects may occur in rare cases. These side effects include skin irritation, redness, itching, or allergic reactions in some sensitive people. To check for adverse reactions, it is essential to perform a patch test on a small area of skin before using products containing witch hazel.

Contraindications:
Although witch hazel is considered safe for topical use, some contraindications exist. It is not recommended for people with known allergies to witch hazel or its components. Topical use on open wounds or damaged skin should also be avoided, as it may cause additional irritation. It is best to consult a healthcare professional if you are pregnant or nursing.

Interactions:
In general, it has no significant interactions with medications or other herbs. However, it is essential to use caution when using witch hazel products with other topical products to avoid potential adverse effects. Suppose you are using any other topical medications. In that case, it is advisable to speak with a healthcare professional before using products containing this plant to ensure no negative interactions.

FINAL NOTE

Thank you very much for choosing this book to accompany you on your path to complete health. If you find the information, advice, or remedies I share here useful, would you do me a favor? Taking a moment to leave your review or rating (several stars would be greatly appreciated) is an incredible way to help me continue creating valuable content while also guiding others who, like you, are seeking to improve their health and well-being. Thank you so much for being part of this wellness community!

With gratitude,

Isabel

Important Note on Printing and Shipping:
All of my paperback books are printed and distributed exclusively by Amazon and its affiliated printing facilities. If you encounter any issues with print quality or delivery, please contact Amazon Customer Service directly for assistance.

As the author, I have no control over these processes, so I kindly request that your reviews focus solely on the content, remedies, or information within this work. Some readers leave negative ratings due to shipping or binding issues, unaware that these matters are, unfortunately, entirely beyond my control and ability to resolve. Thank you from the bottom of my heart for your understanding!

AUTHOR'S BOOKS

▸ **ACID REFLUX.** Foods, Supplements & Medicinal Plants
▸ **ALLERGIES.** Foods, Supplements & Herbs
▸ **ANXIETY.** Foods, Supplements & Herbs
▸ **ARTHRITIS.** Foods, Supplements & Medicinal Plants
▸ **CHOLESTEROL.** Foods, Supplements & Medicinal Plants
▸ **DIABETES.** Foods, Supplements & Herbs
▸ **CONSTIPATION.** Foods, Supplements & Herbs
▸ **FIBROMYALGIA.** Foods, Supplements & Medicinal Plants
▸ **GASTRITIS.** Foods, Supplements & Herbs
▸ **HEMORRHOIDS.** Foods, Supplements & Herbs
▸ **HYPERTENSION.** Foods, Supplements & Medicinal Plants
▸ **INSOMNIA.** Foods, Supplements & Herbs
▸ **MENOPAUSE.** Foods, Supplements & Medicinal Plants
▸ **OSTEOARTHRITIS.** Foods, Supplements & Herbs
▸ **SIBO.** Foods, Supplements & Medicinal Plants
▸ **VARICOSE VEINS.** Foods, Supplements & Herbs

Roots that Inspire: From Obstacles to New Horizons

Born in 1971 in Gáldar, Gran Canaria, Isabel grew up in an environment steeped in tradition and ancestral wisdom. Surrounded by the knowledge of her homeland, she learned from an early age to appreciate the healing power of medicinal plants, home remedies, and the importance of nutrition as foundations for nurturing both body and soul. This heritage, passed down through generations, shaped her childhood and sparked a deep passion for natural medicine—a passion that would eventually become the guiding force of her life.

The journey, however, was not without obstacles. In her youth, Isabel faced a period of profound difficulty: after her separation, she embraced the sole responsibility of raising her daughters. These were challenging times, with motherhood pushing her to her limits while simultaneously fueling her determination to persevere. Even during moments of uncertainty, she remained steadfast, drawing strength from her unwavering commitment to her values and her profound connection to natural health, which always served as her refuge and inspiration.

Rather than yielding to adversity, Isabel channeled it into a drive for learning and growth. She dedicated countless hours to studying books on medicinal plants, exploring new healing methods, and deepening her knowledge of natural remedies. Over the years, she pursued extensive training in naturopathy, nutrition, and complementary therapies, often sacrificing personal comforts to follow her passion. Her dedication not only provided for her family but also enabled her to profoundly impact the lives of those who sought her guidance. People came to trust her wisdom, turning to her for advice and support, and her efforts ignited transformations in countless lives.

A pivotal moment came in the 1990s when she made the decision to professionalize her calling. She embarked on formal training as a naturopath and therapist specializing in alternative health practices. This step was transformative, opening new doors and broadening her ability to serve others. Her expertise, combined with her authentic desire to help, allowed her to support a growing community of people. Every story of healing and recovery deepened her sense of purpose, and she rebuilt her life around her mission to uplift others.

But Isabel's hunger for knowledge and her desire to inspire others extended beyond her immediate community. In 2017, she took a bold new step: she began to write with the aim of sharing her hard-earned experiences and knowledge on a larger scale. Her books, written in an accessible and heartfelt style, are both informative and empowering. They seamlessly blend practical advice, recipes, and natural health alternatives, inspiring readers to embrace healthier, more balanced lifestyles. Every page radiates her warmth and passion, inviting readers to find solutions for their well-being from within and aligning them to the wisdom of nature.

Today, Isabel's work resonates with countless individuals, especially those seeking to regain their health or reconnect with a more intentional way of living. Her story stands as a powerful reminder that even the greatest challenges can lead to profound purpose. Through resilience and perseverance, she has not only transformed her own life but also paved the way for others to rediscover their harmony with nature and with themselves. Her legacy serves as a celebration of living in balance with the natural world and honoring the deep, inherent connection between humanity and the Earth—a testament that obstacles can be the stepping stones to new horizons and an invitation to care for our body, mind, and planet with respect, awareness, and love.

BIBLIOGRAPHY & SCIENTIFIC STUDIES

1. "Plantas Medicinales de uso en España" - Font Quer, P.
2. "The Essential Guide to Herbal Safety" - Simon Mills y Kerry Bone.
3. "Herbal Medicine: Biomolecular and Clinical Aspects" - Iris F. F. Benzie y Sissi Wachtel-Galor.
4. "The Complete Herbal Tutor: The Definitive Guide to the Principles and Practices of Herbal Medicine" - Anne McIntyre.
5. "Encyclopedia of Herbal Medicine" - Andrew Chevallier.
6. "Herbal Remedies" - Andrew Chevallier.
7. "The Earthwise Herbal: A Complete Guide to Old World Medicinal Plants" - Matthew Wood.
8. "Guía de las plantas medicinales" - Lesley Bremness.
9. "Materia Médica Vegetal" - Jorge Alonso.
10. "The Modern Herbal Dispensatory: A Medicine-Making Guide" - Thomas Easley y Steven Horne.
11. "Plantas Medicinales en la Amazonía Peruana: Realidad y Perspectivas" - Luis Delgado y Rodolfo Vásquez.
12. "The Green Pharmacy: New Discoveries in Herbal Remedies for Common Diseases and Conditions" - James A. Duke.
13. "Healing Herbal Teas: Learn to Blend 101 Specially Formulated Teas for Stress Management, Common Ailments & More" - Sarah Farr.
14. "Herbal Antivirals: Natural Remedies for Emerging & Resistant Viral Infections" - Stephen Harrod Buhner.
15. "Medicinal Plants of the World: Chemical Constituents, Traditional and Modern Medicinal Uses" - Ivan A. Ross.
16. "Phytotherapy Desk Reference" - Kerry Bone.
17. "A Modern Herbal" - Mrs. M. Grieve.
18. "Plantas Medicinales: La realidad de una tradición milenaria" - Francisco Javier García Bacca.
19. "The Herbal Handbook: A User's Guide to Medical Herbalism" - David Hoffmann.
20. "Plantas medicinales: El Dioscórides renovado" - Pius Font i Quer.

SCIENTIFIC STUDIES
1. "Topical application of Aloe vera for the treatment of acute and chronic hemorrhoids" - Dabur Research Foundation.

2. "The efficacy of Aloe vera gel in the treatment of first and

second-degree hemorrhoids: a randomized controlled trial" - Koochek, A., et al.

3. "Aloe vera: A short review" - Surjushe, A., et al.

4. "Bilberry (Vaccinium myrtillus) in the treatment of chronic venous insufficiency and hemorrhoids" - Canter, P. H., et al.

5. "The clinical applications of Vaccinium myrtillus (bilberry) in ophthalmology and beyond" - Zafra-Stone, S., et al.

6. "Therapeutic applications of Vaccinium myrtillus (bilberry) for the treatment of hemorrhoids" - Basu, A., et al.

7. "Horse chestnut seed extract for chronic venous insufficiency" - Pittler, M. H., et al.

8. "The effectiveness of Aesculus hippocastanum (horse chestnut) for the treatment of chronic venous insufficiency" - Sirtori, C. R.

9. "Horse chestnut seed extract for venous insufficiency and hemorrhoids" - Siebert, U., et al.

10. "Effect of psyllium hydrophilic mucilloid on constipation and hemorrhoids during pregnancy" - Fernandez-Banares, F., et al.

11. "Psyllium husk in the treatment of hemorrhoids: a randomized, controlled study" - McRorie, J. W., et al.

12. "The role of dietary fiber in the treatment of hemorrhoids" - Alonso-Coello, P., et al.

13. "The use of witch hazel (Hamamelis virginiana) extracts for the treatment of hemorrhoids" - Blumenthal, M., et al.

14. "Clinical efficacy of a witch hazel ointment in the management of hemorrhoids: a randomized, controlled trial" - Beer, A. M., et al.

15. "Hamamelis virginiana (witch hazel) and its therapeutic traditional uses for hemorrhoids" - Gruenwald, J., et al.

16. "Omega-3 fatty acids in inflammation and autoimmune diseases" - Simopoulos, A. P.

17. "The role of omega-3 fatty acids in the management of

inflammatory conditions" - Calder, P. C.

18. "Omega-3 fatty acids and their role in the treatment of hemorrhoids" - Kremer, J. M., et al.

19. "Flaxseed (Linum usitatissimum) as a source of polyphenols and fiber for the treatment of hemorrhoids" - Goyal, A., et al.

20. "Therapeutic applications of flaxseed in the management of hemorrhoids" - Prasad, K.

21. "The effects of flaxseed consumption on bowel health and hemorrhoids" - Bloedon, L. T., et al.

22. "Vitamin E in dermatology" - Thiele, J. J., et al.

23. "The role of vitamin E in the treatment of chronic venous insufficiency and hemorrhoids" - Segre, T. V.

24. "Potential benefits of vitamin E in the management of hemorrhoids" - Zingg, J. M., et al.

25. "Ginkgo biloba in the treatment of chronic venous insufficiency and hemorrhoids: a review" - Pittler, M. H., et al.

26. "The effectiveness of Ginkgo biloba extract in the treatment of hemorrhoids" - Kleijnen, J., et al.

27. "The use of Ginkgo biloba for the treatment of hemorrhoids: a systematic review" - Bone, K.

28. "Ginger (Zingiber officinale) in the management of gastrointestinal disorders" - Ali, B. H., et al.

29. "The effects of ginger on gastrointestinal function and its potential use in the treatment of hemorrhoids" - Lete, I., et al.

30. "Ginger for health benefits and its role in the treatment of hemorrhoids" - Mashhadi, N. S., et al.

31. "Chamomile (Matricaria chamomilla) as a therapeutic option for hemorrhoids" - McKay, D. L., et al.

32. "The efficacy of chamomile in the treatment of hemorrhoids: a randomized clinical trial" - Srivastava, J. K., et al.

33. "Chamomile: A herbal medicine of the past with bright

future" - Srivastava, J. K., et al.

34. "Ruscus aculeatus in the treatment of chronic venous insufficiency and hemorrhoids" - Pittler, M. H., et al.

35. "Efficacy of Ruscus aculeatus extract in the management of hemorrhoids" - Michel, P., et al.

36. "Therapeutic efficacy of Ruscus aculeatus in the treatment of hemorrhoids" - Vanscheidt, W., et al.

37. "Red vine leaf extract (Vitis vinifera) for the treatment of chronic venous insufficiency and hemorrhoids" - Belcaro, G., et al.

38. "The role of Vitis vinifera in the management of hemorrhoids" - di Pierro, F., et al.

39. "Clinical applications of red vine leaf extract in the treatment of hemorrhoids" - Kiesewetter, H., et al.

40. "Red vine leaf extract in the treatment of chronic venous insufficiency: a review". Autores: Suter A, Bommer S, Rechner J.